The WEIGHTED BLANKET Guide

Everything You Need to Know about Weighted Blankets
and Deep Pressure for Autism, Chronic Pain,
and Other Conditions

Eileen Parker and Cara Koscinski

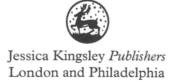

Jessica Kingsley *Publishers*
London and Philadelphia

First published in 2016
by Jessica Kingsley Publishers
73 Collier Street
London N1 9BE, UK
and
400 Market Street, Suite 400
Philadelphia, PA 19106, USA

www.jkp.com

Copyright © Eileen Parker and Cara Koscinski 2016

Printed digitally since 2016

Library of Congress Cataloging in Publication Data
Names: Parker, Eileen, 1966- author. | Koscinski, Cara, author.
Title: The weighted blanket guide : everything you need to know about weighted blankets and deep pressure for autism, chronic pain, and other conditions / Eileen Parker and Cara Koscinski.
Description: London ; Philadelphia : Jessica Kingsley Publishers, 2016. | Includes bibliographical references and index.
Identifiers: LCCN 2015049917 | ISBN 9781849057189 (alk. paper)
Subjects: LCSH: Occupational therapy. | Mind and body therapies.
Classification: LCC RC487 .P37 2016 | DDC 615.8/515--dc23
LC record available at http://lccn.loc.gov/2015049917

British Library Cataloguing in Publication Data
A CIP catalogue record for this book is available from the British Library

ISBN 978 1 84905 718 9
eISBN 978 1 78450 202 7

Z984186

"I am thr[...] [...]nket guide. It answers so many questions that people have about weighted blanket therapy. There is no one more suited to write it than Eileen, a onetime fellow weighted blanket maker and a user of weighted blankets for her own autism."
—Donna Chambers, Founder, SensaCalm Weighted Blankets

"When I was a child, I craved deep pressure and I liked lots of blankets on the bed to help me sleep. When I got older, I built a squeeze machine to apply deep pressure to help calm me. Sensory problems are very variable. A weighted blanket is likely to be most effective for children or adults who seek deep pressure. For children with an autism diagnosis, some individuals will respond well to a weighted blanket and for others it will have little effect. This book contains lots of good practical advice on how to use and make weighted blankets. It will be a great resource for individuals who are calmed by deep pressure."
—Temple Grandin, author of The Autistic Brain and Thinking in Pictures

"Cara Koscinski and Eileen Parker have written the definitive guide to weighted blankets. As an Autism Mom and an individual with fibromyalgia, I wish I'd had this book years ago. I finally understand the symptoms of sensory processing disorder and how pressure can counteract them. I especially love the detailed instructions on how to sew my own weighted blanket, including smart color choices for individuals with autism spectrum disorder. This book is a must for anyone thinking about using a weighted blanket!"
—Shannon Penrod, Host of Autism Live

of related interest

**The Parent's Guide to Occupational Therapy
for Autism and Other Special Needs**
Practical Strategies for Motor Skills, Sensory
Integration, Toilet Training, and More
Cara Koscinski
ISBN 978 1 78592 705 8
eISBN 978 1 78450 258 4

**An Occupational Therapist's Guide
to Sleep and Sleep Problems**
Edited by Andrew Green and Cary Brown
ISBN 978 1 84905 618 2
eISBN 978 1 78450 088 7

The Mystery of Pain
Douglas Nelson
ISBN 978 1 84819 152 5
eISBN 978 0 85701 116 9

Can I tell you about Sensory Processing Difficulties?
A guide for friends, family and professionals
Sue Allen
Illustrated by Mike Medaglia
Part of the *Can I tell you about...?* Series
ISBN 978 1 84905 640 3
eISBN 978 1 78450 137 2

Disclaimer

Every effort has been made to provide up-to-date, unbiased, and accurate information. No information contained herein is a substitute for medical advice obtained by your physician.

Neither the authors nor the publisher take responsibility for any consequences of any decision made as a result of the information contained in this book.

REMEMBER

- Never wrap someone up in a weighted blanket. It should always be placed on top of the user, who should be able to remove it easily.

- Always use the lowest amount of weight possible that still achieves therapeutic benefits. Ask your occupational therapist or medical professional for advice.

- Weighted blankets will not necessarily work for everyone. Like all therapeutic tools, it is worth trying them to see if they are effective for you.

- Temple Grandin reminded Cara that her squeeze machines are equipped with a "dead man's switch" so that if the user becomes incapacitated or unable to independently pull the lever, the machine releases all pressure. It is critical to provide users of weighted blankets this same safety measure. This can be achieved by ensuring that the blankets are not used on anyone who cannot remove the blanket independently. We are often asked if the blankets should be used on those who are cognitively unable to remove the blanket and the answer is always, "No."

Contents

About the Authors   9

Acknowledgments   11

Chapter 1   Introducing Weighted Blankets   13
    What is a weighted blanket?   13
    What are they used for?   14
       Sleep   17
       Chronic pain and fibromyalgia   20
       Anxiety   23
       Autism   23
       Alzheimer's/dementia/seniors   24
       Mental illnesses   25
       Special education   28

Chapter 2   Where Did the Concept Come From?   31
    The old meeting the new   31
    Others' stories   32
    Origins   34

Chapter 3   How Weighted Blankets Work   37
    Your sensory system   38
    What problems result from SPD?   45
    Exploring deep pressure   48

Massage   49

Neuroscience   52

Chapter 4   Professional Settings   59

Occupational therapy   59

   What is occupational therapy?   59

   How are weighted blankets used at an OT clinic?   61

   How does OT work for SPD?   62

Hospital use   65

   Restraint reduction   66

   Actual use in a hospital setting   71

Comfort/multisensory rooms   73

Helping patients getting weighted blankets covered
by medical insurance   75

Chapter 5   Considerations/Guidelines
for Use   77

   Can they create dependence?   77

   How long to use the blanket?   78

   Safety   79

   Drawbacks/concerns   80

   Medical insurance coverage   82

Chapter 6   Choosing or Making Your Own   87

   Choosing a weighted blanket   87

   On a budget   95

   Sewing your own weighted blanket   96

Postscript   103

References   105

Index   109

About the Authors

Eileen Parker has autism and sensory processing disorder. She first tried a weighted blanket at occupational therapy, which led to her owning a weighted blanket company for six years. In this book, she will give her personal experiences and her knowledge learned through her business. She sleeps with a 34-pound queen-size on her bed. "I" throughout the book refers to Eileen.

Pediatric occupational therapist Cara Koscinski, MOT, OTR/L, known as *The Pocket Occupational Therapist*, is an author of numerous books on occupational therapy and autism, a frequent magazine contributor, and a national speaker. She has successfully founded two pediatric therapy clinics and has created CDs for children with autism and auditory sensitivity. Her two children have autism, so she knows how much their weighted blankets help them.

Acknowledgments

Eileen
Thank you to John, who supported me through writing this book. Thanks to my mum, who for years has been telling me to write for a living, because after all, Mother knows best. And thank you Jane Evans at Jessica Kingsley Publishers and Cara for your enthusiasm for this book.

Cara
To those near and dear to me in the occupational therapy field—your support lifts me daily and fills me with excitement for our profession. Nicole LaRose, your enthusiasm for occupational therapy and for helping my lil guy live a better life brings me to tears. Sue at Clap Your Hands, my boys *love* their weighted blankets. You are a blessing! To all of my clients—working with you pushes me to be better every day. Jessica Kingsley Publishers, thank you for believing in our book. Eileen, I've so enjoyed your passion for weighted blankets and desire to deliver quality information that is accessible to everyone.

Chapter 1

Introducing
Weighted Blankets

What is a weighted blanket?

In its simplest form, a weighted blanket is two pieces of fabric sewn together with a heavy filling inside. The filling is sewn into squares to give even weight distribution. From that simple method, a new generation of weighted blanket makers have grown up, a whole industry built around this "new" concept of weight on the body.

Many liken a weighted blanket to the feeling of the lead vest at the dentist's office. A weighted blanket can give that same feeling, but better because the blanket is pliable to give a feeling of an overall big hug. The material which is added to provide the blanket's weight offers conforming comfort to the user.

Think about weighted blankets differently than you would a regular blanket. They are not about keeping warm, rather about the weight on the body. While most weighted blankets on the market aren't designed for warmth, some blankets have batting in them to give warmth as a comforter would.

While weighted blankets are not a "cure for all ills," some feel they help tremendously. The benefits can often occur immediately after donning the blanket. The medical community is adopting them rapidly to help patients calm and regulate themselves and sleep better. They are so effective, some medical insurance plans in the U.S. cover them when prescribed by a professional.

What are they used for?

A 2008 study by Mullen *et al.* on the effects of weighted blanket use in adults found that some participants reported decreased anxiety and felt more relaxed.

We conducted a survey of over 300 occupational therapists (OTs) (Parker n.d.). They reported that patients with the following conditions had improvement with the use of weighted blankets. I have also included conditions helped that I learned of while at my weighted blanket company:

- sensory processing disorder (SPD)

- autism

- stress/anxiety

- post-traumatic stress disorder (PTSD)

- traumatic brain injury (TBI)

- chronic pain

- major mental illness

- insomnia

- restless legs syndrome (RLS)

- Alzheimer's/dementia

- chemotherapy

- post-surgery

- motor agitation

- attention deficit hyperactivity disorder (ADHD)
- cerebral palsy
- substance/alcohol detoxing
- Rett syndrome
- multiple sclerosis
- fetal alcohol syndrome (FAS)
- apraxia
- fibromyalgia.

As a former weighted blanket company owner, I know how these blankets help people to different degrees. I use the disclaimer "Individual results will vary" because the benefit received depends on the individual. Some people feel the effects immediately, and if a client doesn't report positive results after three nights of use, I usually consider increasing the weight of the blanket.

Parents who ordered weighted blankets often reported that their child slept the "best ever" from the first night the blanket was used. For some individuals, it took several nights to notice an effect.

It has made a significant difference for me, a person with autism and co-occurring sensory processing disorder. I first tried a weighted blanket while I was receiving sensory integration therapy at my local occupational therapy clinic. My occupational therapist, Suzie, had me lie down on a gym mat then she put the blanket on me. It immediately felt "weird" and the effect started in seconds. It felt like my muscles were melting down into the mat. But the blanket was denim, so it felt scratchy and the ends where they were sewn were hard and rubbed under my chin. I like a much softer blanket, but others may love the denim.

Like most other people, sleep and anxiety are the main reasons I use a weighted blanket. It makes me feel calm and sleepy. My anxiety goes down and my brain slows from its constant chatter. I feel safer.

People with autism are the largest consumers of weighted blankets since they usually have a co-occurring sensory processing disorder and insomnia. The weighted blankets help them to calm themselves and to get much-needed sleep, or in the case of children, both the children and the parents get to sleep.

They are so effective that a growing number of hospitals are using them on a variety of units, including post-surgery, mental health, pediatric, geriatric, and others. As of this writing, I have heard of studies on the use of weighted blankets that are underway at hospitals, so if you know someone who is involved in a study, go to the back of the book to contact one of us as we would be interested in the study methods and conclusions.

Some people have found the weighted blanket similar to working on the body's pressure points which they experience in occupational or physical therapy or while receiving deep tissue massage.

So many have found relief from chronic pain, such as fibromyalgia, yet the reason is unknown. Even though comprehensive studies will be needed to understand the effects of weighted blankets, I will address possible reasons in a later chapter.

Weighted blankets are also a tremendous help for post-traumatic stress disorder. While in its infancy, some therapists at counseling centers use them for their clients in-session since PTSD can raise such intense emotion and stress. The blanket helps them to feel grounded and in the moment so they are better at dealing with the emotions, and can "come down" from the intensity.

During the course of working with the public at my former weighted blanket business, countless numbers of people inquired about the blankets. This commonly occurred online or even in a queue at the post office. I explained who they are used for (autistic people, people on mental health units at hospitals, special education students, jail inmates, etc.), but the first assumption was often that the blankets may have been designed to restrain a person. I was quick to explain that the blanket is utilized for comforting people, lowering anxiety, and getting to sleep and staying asleep. They were usually amazed and curious, and yes, I gave them my card. Inevitably they said that it was so nice I was helping people.

Sleep

A study in the U.K. found that weighted blankets do not help with sleep in children with autism (Gringras *et al.* 2014). There is no study proving the blankets help with sleep, but there is much anecdotal evidence—especially client and caregiver reports. Also, in our own questionnaire of OTs, sleep improvement was reported by 64.6 percent. Gringras *et al.*'s study results were documented in *Pediatrics*, the official journal of the American Academy of Pediatrics:

> Seventy-three children were randomized and analysis conducted on 67 children who completed the study. Using objective measures, the weighted blanket, compared with the control blanket, did not increase TST [total sleep time] as measured by actigraphy and adjusted for baseline TST.

(Actigraphy is a method of recording rest and activity cycles. An actigraph unit, worn on the wrist, records movement, which can give information to researchers on the subject's sleep patterns at home. Researchers can use this to record a baseline before multiple types of recording in a clinical setting.)

They found no difference in the quantity or quality of sleep, falling asleep faster, or waking less often, but subjectively the parents and children preferred the weighted blanket.

In the survey we conducted with 303 OTs, they reported that people were calmer with reduced anxiety (90.4%), better able to control behavior (47.5%), had increased focus/were more aware of surroundings (55.7%), slept better (64.6%), or showed no difference (9.3%).

As a person with autism, my issues with sleep are not unusual.

I remember growing up that I would roll myself in my comforter to try to feel "tight." The greater the pressure I felt from rolling myself up, the better I felt, and the better I slept. If I couldn't get it tight enough, I would get frustrated and keep trying to get it to just the right tightness.

If I woke up in the night to use the bathroom, I would repeat the whole process all over again.

Even with all that, it still didn't feel tight enough. It felt like my body was light and airy—unprotected perhaps. I would lie there trying to get to sleep feeling like I was on hyper-alert. The street light shone in my window onto the angled ceiling over my bed. I would lie there following the wallpaper patterns over and over again. I could never visually reconcile the edges of the wallpaper that didn't perfectly line up with the next piece of wallpaper.

I now sleep with a queen-size weighted blanket on my bed and I have a 15-pound throw on my couch—and no wallpaper.

Here are comments from others about sleep:

The [weighted blanket] is already working. It is amazing how Elizabeth settles right down to go to sleep! It is already worth its weight in gold. Thank you so much.

—Susan

I meant to send this a while ago, but thank you so much for the blanket! It has helped with my insomnia more than I ever imagined. I'm no longer tossing and turning at night, waking up countless times, or having trouble getting to sleep. Even when I only have time for a few hours or even a nap, I feel so refreshed afterwards. Now I found a new problem though—I never want to get out of bed in the morning!!

—Katie

Thank you so much for the weighted blanket. It's been the answer we were looking for. My son is 12 and had never slept through the night prior to getting this blanket. We ordered this blanket hoping that this might work as I noticed my son liked to sleep under heavy pillows. From the first night, my son has not had any more sleep issues. He loves the blanket and sleeps soundly in his room. He even took the blanket with him on a sleepover to a friend's house. The blanket is soft and warm, and washes easily. Thank you again, my son now sleeps through the night. I only wish I had known about the blanket sooner.

—Kim

I have had difficulty sleeping for about ten years. I have usually taken a medication to sleep. I tried using a weighted blanket and found that it had similar effects but without the medication. I was able to feel relaxed and drowsy, which helped me to fall asleep. I slept soundly through the night and I am no longer worried about falling asleep or having to take medication to fall asleep.

—Julie

I wanted to let you know that I ordered a blanket for my daughter a while back, and it is amazing. She started having a hard time sleeping when her new baby brother arrived. We had taken her to a sleep specialist, with very little relief. The blanket did the trick. We now get ten wonderful hours of sleep every night. Thank you so much!

—Sarah

The blanket arrived yesterday. I love it!!! It looks great but it feels amazing. Who knew? All these years I spent piling on blankets to create weight. I had the best night's sleep ever.

—Nancy

We ordered our son's weighted blanket...and he just loves his blanket; so do we, because he sleeps better at night.

—Whitney

Chronic pain and fibromyalgia

This section is partially based on an interview with Doug Nelson, author of *The Mystery of Pain*.

A possible reason why weighted blankets may work is developing from research on our outside senses. Touch gives us a feedback mechanism from our own sensory map, which quiets the insula, also known as the insular cortex. (The insular cortex is the part of the brain involved with sensation, subjective feelings, perception, interpersonal experience, self-awareness, motor control, empathy, and more. Body functions known as interoceptive awareness are regulated by the insula. An interoceptor is a specialized sensory nerve receptor that receives and responds to stimuli originating from within the body.)

The insula is a part of the brain whose functions are only just being discovered. It quiets the central nervous system (CNS) with postsynaptic inhibition, which then quiets the pain sensation. The feedback mechanism through touch may explain why massage or hands on the body makes the CNS remap itself. A weighted blanket may share some of the same mechanisms, but different, by quieting in a way that massage can't do.

Nelson says, "As with fibromyalgia, the peripheral nervous system is overly lit up or overexcited." According to the National Cancer Institute (2015), the peripheral nervous system "consists of the nerves that branch out from the brain and spinal cord. These nerves form the communication network between the CNS and the body parts."

Nelson continues:

> Putting hands on a person with fibromyalgia through massage or touch can be an added stimulus that is one too many, since the brain processes it as a novelty, an added stimulus, but the weighted blanket would be comforting since it is constant pressure that would override the feeling with a comforting neurofeedback mechanism.

When I had my weighted blanket company, so many people reported relief from chronic pain by using a weighted blanket, such as for fibromyalgia. The controversy around the existence of fibromyalgia rages on since it is something that is felt, not seen. Ditto for a weighted blanket. How can something that is not a pill or a pin prick help so much? But this is what people have written to me:

> *I have fibromyalgia, rheumatoid arthritis and restless legs syndrome and I saw an ad for this in a fibromyalgia magazine and thought I'd give it a try, but I have to admit I was a little skeptical about paying that much for something I wasn't sure about. I'm taking so much medicine, that I wanted to try something else.*

After reading some articles and reviews, I decided to order. Boy, am I ever glad I did! ... I can't really figure out why and how it works, but I don't care—it truly relieves pain for me. When I'm having a bad day, I lie on the couch and pull my "blankie" over me and I immediately start feeling better psychologically because I know that soon I'm either going to start feeling better physically and/or I'm going to fall peacefully asleep.

The best thing about it is the pain relief that I get from this blanket. I can't really explain it, except to say that maybe it calms the nerves that I feel are going crazy under my skin. Another benefit is the relaxation effect—I always fall asleep! I have even tried to stay awake just as a test, but I can't do it. Even though it sounds heavy, it really isn't uncomfortable at all since it's spread out...

Another thing I was concerned about was that it would be too hot, but somehow it's not at all. It's the best thing I've done for myself in a long time!

I don't want to ever have to be without it!

—Barb

I don't like taking pills. One less pill, the better. I don't know if I'm going to refill my prescription for my RLS [restless legs syndrome], because I put my [blanket company name] blanket on at night. Normally, I wake up from the rustling around my legs, but I don't wake up anymore. It saves me money, and it's one less pill to take.

—Melanie

When my muscles are jumpy and achy from the fibro, I love curling up with mine!!

—Rachel

Anxiety

I experience anxiety, some of it from having autism and SPD, and a great deal from PTSD, so managing it is important for my daily functioning. With my PTSD, when I am experiencing symptoms, my body and mind feel raw and exposed. I feel out of control and have the fight-or-flight response. For all three of these conditions, the weighted blanket helps me. When I am triggered by an event that reminds me of the trauma, I seek my weighted blanket on the couch, and as is common with autism, I rock my body.

> *I have to buy another weighted blanket because my daughter stole mine and won't give it back. It's the best stress reducer and relaxation aid ever!*
>
> —Pam

Autism

By far, most weighted blankets are used for people with autism. Caregivers and professionals in the autism community have a great awareness of their benefits, including feeling more secure, improving feeling of body awareness, reducing anxiety, and improving sleep. Occupational therapists frequently recommend the blankets for their clients in order to help calm and stimulate the tactile receptors.

Autism can be stressful because we encounter situations where we don't have the skills or the brain type to handle them. Sometimes, it's the feeling of rejection from others or being the one left out of conversations or situations that can cause anxiety, anger, sadness, or other extreme emotions. Sometimes it's simply a change of routine that can cause an extreme out-of-control feeling.

With sensory processing disorder, which almost always occurs with autism, sensory messages aren't processed correctly by the brain. Other people can focus on one sound and "not notice" the rest, but for a person with SPD, *all* the signals come in and aren't processed correctly, which creates an overload and makes me feel like screaming and running away.

According to the Sensory Processing Disorder Foundation's website, more than three-quarters of children with autism also have sensory processing disorder. It is common for those with autism to be under-responsive, needing more stimuli to achieve regulation of the body. The opposite is true as well—some individuals with autism may be over-responsive or require a calm environment to function optimally. They tend to be unable to get used to, or habituate to, information such as noise, touch, smell, etc.

My son's weighted blanket is sure a blessing!! He has autism and therefore sleeping problems as well as typical meltdowns. After having it a few months he has become as attached to it as he is his own favorite blanket. It still calms meltdowns, great for sensory breaks, and he just falls asleep so much better than he ever has...and I will tell everyone I know how well the blanket works!

—Lisa

Alzheimer's/dementia/seniors

I interviewed Tresha Melquist, Director of Nursing for Long Term Care at Cokato Charitable Trust, of which their nursing home part is Cokato Manor in Cokato, Minnesota. They do long-term care, some short-term rehab, and some mobility and dementia services.

For wandering, we used to have alarms, which was startling to the residents so we got rid of them for the dignity factor. We wanted to find something to give them comfort, so we give one to residents so it becomes their blanket. We have found them to be very effective.

We did a couple of trials. If they are very restless or appear afraid, we drape a small blanket over their shoulders so it feels like someone is there with them. They appear more calm, and it seems like they are more content and not as restless and anxious. We have a couple of residents who use them when they are more anxious, usually people with more advanced dementia.

We are getting away from restraints, such as tying them to a chair so they don't fall. We now use the weighted blanket which gives them nice pressure, and it comforts them so they aren't getting up from the wheelchair and falling.

She says that if they have a hard time getting to sleep, a weighted blanket makes them feel like someone is hugging, and it's a positive pressure that is more comforting to them. People with dementia often have a poor sleep pattern, but the weighted blanket definitely helps them sleep and helps to keep them in bed longer.

Mental illnesses

Weighted blankets are increasingly being used in behavioural health (mental health) units so patients can soothe themselves.

A patient presenting with bipolar I disorder and comorbid anxiety, ADHD, and dyslexia was taught deep touch pressure strategies to alleviate severe symptoms of sensory over-responsivity and anxiety. The patient reported that the techniques were helpful as they allowed her to cope with potentially overwhelming situations in her environment. Clinician-rated functioning also improved over the course of treatment. This case study suggests that deep touch pressure may be useful in patients with bipolar disorder who have SOR (sensory over-responsivity) and anxiety as comorbid conditions. (Sylvia *et al.* 2014)

Gretchen Prohofsky, BH Allied Health Manager at Regions Hospital, reported that since they began using weighted blankets on their inpatient mental health units, they saw a drastic decline in the use of seclusion and restraint, as well as safety sitters. (Safety sitters are professionals who stay with the patient to prevent suicide or overdosing, or to avoid the use of restraints. The primary job of a safety sitter is to keep a patient safe. Sometimes a safety sitter is called a "one-on-one.") Prohofsky reported that many patients who used the blankets feel calmer, more grounded, safe and secure, centered, with improved concentration and decreased stress and anxiety, as well as having improved sleep. Throughout our own research, we have found a great deal of consistency in this area. Prohofsky said:

> The patients are very interested in learning about their sensory processing disorder and request reading materials to increase their understanding. The patients are also receptive to utilizing additional sensory tools to positively impact their quality of life... The weighted blankets are working miracles! (personal communication, 2014)

Remember that self-regulation skills assist us in regulating our emotions and general sense of "well-being." Maintaining an appropriate level of alertness, processing sensory information we receive through our senses, and demonstrating the ability to organize and plan give us a uniqueness that sets us apart from other animals. Our self-regulation includes our own emotions and past experiences. We maintain our own body rhythms in order to function in day-to-day life. When we sleep or wake, how we move (transition) from task to task, and our ability to "cheer ourselves up" when we feel down are all examples of self-regulation tasks. Oftentimes, when someone lives with a disability, they may experience difficulty with self-regulation.

I interviewed OT Angie Balzarini Leonhart, who is the sensory specialist at Regions Hospital.

> I have observed that the deep pressure is helpful for patients. They start to relax, their muscle tone relaxes, they make increased eye contact and, when their speech is anxiously rapid, their speech slows down. They have a general look of physical relief.

She says patients report that they feel comfortable, less anxious, and as though they are receiving a "hug." It is common for patients to report feeling less agitated and calmer. When considering the use of weighted blankets in clinics such as Regions Hospital, it's important to be careful when patients are in a psychotic state, which is not the appropriate time to introduce the blankets. Patients must be aware of the blanket's use and must understand how to use it when they need to calm themselves. Leonhart continues:

> Number one, we are able to identify the red flags, the indicators that they may have sensory issues such as anxiety, chemical dependency, trauma, BPD (borderline personality disorder), or self-injury. With trauma, they usually have very fragile nervous systems, which is a higher indicator for sensory issues.
>
> Many patients are receptive initially because they want to try different sensory interventions. After they have tried sensory methods, they automatically know what they need, like a fidget, headphones, or a weighted blanket. Many times, OTs do a sensory consultation

screen, which helps to determine what interventions are helpful and soothing, Additionally, practitioners are constantly seeking ways of funding the blankets so the patients have more resources.

There is no scientific proof that weighted blankets work. But, a great deal of anecdotal evidence supports that they do work. Since they *do* work for so many, why? Is it the placebo effect? It is realistic to assume that there are likely reasons we don't even know yet.

Special education

Weighted blankets are a staple in most special education classrooms. They are often used in a "quiet room" where the student can relax from being "wound up," anxious, or stressed. Sometimes while working, the student will have a weighted lap pad or neck wrap to keep their anxiety down. The blanket calms them down so they can focus and do their work. Teachers report that students seek them when things overwhelm them.

> *Typically, I suggest using weighted blankets during seated tasks or where focus/control is expected and then remove the blanket after the task is completed. Pairing tasks which require focus with tactile and proprioceptive input can help to improve self-regulation.*
>
> *—from OT survey*

> *Weighted blankets are a fantastic way to calm an anxious or jumpy child. We use the lap [pads] all day long with students who come in our room to work on tests, homework or just take a break. Not only does it calm them, but my data has shown that they are more productive and can focus for longer intervals. Also we teachers will often drape them around our shoulders to ease tension. It's a great stress relief for everyone.*

Even my giant dog uses the big full-size weighted blanket during thunderstorms to help calm his nerves.

—Melanie, special education teacher

I recommend this kind of weighted blanket for special ed classrooms. It helps them concentrate and focus.

—Kristin, special education teacher

I am a previous special education teacher and I know so many children who could benefit from these. They are less stigmatizing than the weighted medicaid vests that scream look at me…there's something wrong…again, love mine!!

—Laura, special education teacher

I have observed that they have a sense of calming, security, quietness, and relaxation. The kids ask for it, and when they are stressed, whether on the [autism] spectrum or not, they know it's here so they can use it.

They lie on the floor or sit at a desk. They like knowing it's here when they feel a need for it. The parents know it's here, and they know that when the student is on sensory overload and wired, it gives them calm and a reset of their mind.

I have them use it when they are overloaded, in conflict with another kid, or frustrated. I have them use it in any situation where a hug would help, but they don't want touch, but the blanket gives them a long-term hug. They use it when they need to get settled in and think about things. It's a self-care, self-directed calming time.

I recommend that other teachers have one available. Teachers tend to have it in elementary schools more because young kids do not have the coping systems like the older ones do. I also have it available to borrow.

This will work for adults also, because it's not just for kids, so they can use one when they need a support to level out and feel calmed.

—Suzanne, special education teacher

Chapter 2

Where Did the Concept Come From?

The old meeting the new

A heavy blanket on the body is not a new concept. In the old days, heavy quilts made of layers of fabric helped many a child sleep.

Here is my experience: I lay on my side in what used to be Uncle Marvin's room, with no streetlights, looking at the total blackness outside. I cuddled up in the quilt Granny made and listened to the crickets through the open window. The light from the kitchen angled into the room that carried Granny and Papa's Finnish voices with it.

The hug of the heavy quilt won over the child's want to stay awake, into dream with memories of all the aunts and uncles sewn into it.

Now that I'm grown, I'm still a kid to Granny, I expect. Quilts have changed since those days and gone with them are the comfort and feeling of safety the old-fashioned country quilts gave me.

You see, quilts from earlier days were made from fabric from clothes no longer needed. They were cut and sewn into squares for the top and had many layers of fabric underneath, which made them quite heavy. Yarn was pulled through the fabric at intervals, and tied to hold the blanket layers together.

I think the yarn on Granny's quilt was red or pink which contrasted nicely with the mostly blue and green patterns in the quilt. I noticed these things, but it was the weight of the quilt that made me feel secure and grounded and safe.

That is my first memory of a weighted blanket, long before it was a new invention.

The quilts these days are made with a light polyester or cotton batting in between the top and bottom layers, so they don't give the hugging feeling like traditional quilt-making did. Now, a new generation of blanket makers has grown up who make weighted blankets. There is a whole industry built around the "new" concept of weight on the body. Hospitals are adopting them rapidly. For some conditions, some medical insurance plans will even cover them as a necessary piece of medical equipment.

Back when heavy quilts were made, a doctor didn't write a prescription, but knowingly or not, Granny at her sewing machine made good medicine.

Others' stories

The inclusion of others' stories is important to us, as much of the evidence that weighted blankets work is evident in the stories of those who use them.

In my childhood we slept under the old-fashioned, fabric-layered quilts my North Carolina grandmother, Miss Willie, made. They were very soft to the touch as she washed the front and back cover several times before she started the actual quilting. The quilts were quite heavy, not like quilts of today. It was a solid, enveloping, weighing down comfort that made you know that you were in bed to stay put. These quilts wrapped you in a warmth that let you stick your nose out into the biting cold and breathe in deeply. The heaviness also felt like protection from the things in the closet and under the bed.

My favorite quilt is the one she made from the scraps of dresses my mother had made for my sister and me. We can now look at the quilt and see memories of every holiday in our childhood.

—Carol

As a child, I slept under a series of very heavy, homemade quilts that my grandmother made for me. I lived in Iowa where the winters were quite cold, and I remember feeling safe and secure under my quilt. I don't remember feeling cold ever, just secure, as if nothing and nobody could bother or harm me.

Later, when I was six years old, we moved to California, and I held on to my quilt even though the weather didn't warrant it. I just didn't feel comfortable unless I slept under it.

Three years later we moved to Arizona, and I was forced to give it up. I felt naked without my quilt and had trouble sleeping for months. It wasn't a child's desire to have a favorite blanket, because I had several different quilts made for me by my grandmother and traded them out without any problem. It was the loss of the weight of the blanket that I remember most. The weight of it made me feel as if nothing could touch me, not little critters like spiders or pests like mosquitoes, and not the monster I sometimes thought lived under my bed.

I felt protected under my heavy quilt, and I still miss that feeling today, even though I'm in my 40s and haven't had a need for a quilt in almost 30 years.

—Beth

I'm 56 years old, so overnight visits at my grandmother's house almost always involved these old heavy quilts. In both summer and winter, they were laid on the floor to make pallets for the grandkids to sleep on. In the winter time, there were more quilts piled on top to keep us warm in a house that had

only two gas heaters—neither of which was left burning at
night. Grandma actually had a huge built-in chest in her
storage/sewing/canned foods room that was specifically built
to store all her quilts.

They were definitely heavy, which made me feel protected
and safe—especially important for a little girl who was afraid
of the dark. One of my all-time favorite memories is waking
up under those layers of delicious warmth to the smell of
coffee and the low murmur of the grown-ups talking at the
kitchen table. My little nose would be cold, but the rest of me
was perfectly cozy and I was content to just lie there snuggled
up until the smell of bacon frying lured me out into the chill
of the morning.

—Barb

Origins

The origin of the first weighted blanket is not known. Vast searches in literature, the internet, and published research yield no indication about the first use of the blankets in the medical and mental health setting. What we do know is that in recent years understanding of the role of the proprioceptive system (awareness of one's own body position, motion, and equilibrium) and tactile system (touch sensations of pressure, vibration, movement, temperature, and pain) has developed markedly, and with this understanding the use of weighted blankets has grown.

One of the most well-known individuals with autism is Dr. Temple Grandin, autism advocate, inventor, and namesake for a major motion picture about her life. As a girl, Temple found and tried a squeeze machine for cattle. While in the machine, she noted relaxing benefits for her own body. She proceeded to note similarities between anxiety in cattle and in individuals with autism.

After years of dedicated research and work with animals, Temple invented ways better to calm them. Additionally, Dr. Grandin invented her own "squeeze machine," which is manufactured by Therafin Corporation today. Users set the appropriate pressure and control when the squeeze is applied. One of the huge benefits of providing deep pressure with the squeeze machine is that the individual has control of when and how often the squeeze is delivered.

Dr. Grandin wrote: "When I built my squeeze machine and Tom McKean made his pressure suits, we did not realize that we were inventing a therapy method that has now helped many children." McKean's pressure suit consisted of a life jacket with a tight scuba suit on top. The valve on the life jacket is used to increase or decrease the feeling of pressure. Decades later, so many are thankful for their discoveries. Weighted blankets and their effect on the tactile receptors provide similar benefits and the positive results described by those who use them.

Chapter 3

How Weighted
Blankets Work

Often when people experience a dysfunction in cognition, PTSD, sensory processing, or many other medical and mental health conditions, they benefit from weighted blankets. Research is still being done to determine the exact reason *why* the blankets work. We will discuss various possibilities here and provide critical information to aid in understanding weighted blankets and sensory processing.

At trade shows, we encouraged people to try out our weighted blankets in a recliner. Many had never tried, or even heard of, a weighted blanket. Once the blanket was on, many responded (often immediately or within a few minutes) with how amazing, relaxed, and sleepy they felt. Very often, the person trying the blanket said to a friend: "You have got to try this. It's amazing!"

Weighted blankets have been in use for many years for individuals who have autism and sensory processing disorders. They have learned of the benefits of blankets through word of mouth, articles, web searches, and by other means. For those who benefit from their use, no specific research is needed. If something works to regulate or show benefit for someone, then no other proof is needed for the individual. Here's an example: Ginger tea or soda

THE WEIGHTED BLANKET GUIDE

is often Grandma's choice for helping a child with a cold. No studies prove that it helps with a cold, but studies have shown conclusive evidence that ginger has antibacterial properties, cancer-fighting properties, and many more important uses. Likewise, cloves have long been used for fighting toothaches and research has later reported the benefits of this tried and true remedy.

Oftentimes, an old wives' tale proves to be a real benefit. Parents often used to run to the store to get ginger ale for an ailing child, while its proven benefits existed in a netherworld of folk medicine. It would be reasonable to believe, then, that prior to research studies, internet, and medical publications familial medical beliefs and healing traditions have been passed down through generations with great success. Could the same be true for the use of heavy quilts or a weighted blanket?

At my weighted blanket business, we had fewer than five returns from people who reported no personal benefit or that they didn't prefer pressure on the body. That is a telling number. Again, the evidence is primarily anecdotal. There are those who prefer studies outlining the benefits of a product and others who strongly attest to the wonderful benefits of the blankets. If it's the placebo effect, hail to the weighted blanket! However, we will outline some theories based on bodies of information both anecdotal and scientific.

Your sensory system

In order to understand weighted blankets, we need to discuss how our body processes sensory information. Let's begin by introducing sensory integration (SI) therapy.

Sensory integration was first introduced formally at a lecture in 1963 by Anna Jean Ayres, PhD, OTR. Dr. Ayres was an occupational therapist and developmental psychologist. While working at UCLA Brain Research Institute, she developed theories on SI. It's important to understand the origins of our understanding of the sensory system. According to an article on the Autism Research Institute website:

> Sensory integration is an innate neurobiological process and refers to the integration and interpretation of sensory stimulation from the environment by the brain. In contrast, sensory integrative dysfunction is a disorder in which sensory input is not integrated or organized appropriately in the brain and may produce varying degrees of problems in development, information processing, and behavior. (Hatch-Rasmussen n.d.)

In order to better describe the difficulty so many have with processing sensory information, occupational therapists and many researchers use the term sensory processing disorder, or SPD. The terms sensory processing disorder and sensory integrative dysfunction are sometimes used interchangeably, however.

As we move through our environment, our body works to make sense of the world around us. We are equipped with a sensory system whose job it is to take in, process, and form outcomes in response to our environment. The sensory system works subconsciously and is out of our control. Designed to protect our bodies from danger, the sensory system relies on 'pre-programmed' information and past experiences.

While SPD often affects the entire body, it's important to consider that there are more than the five senses we are most familiar with: sight (visual), hearing (auditory), taste, smell (olfactory), and touch.

Vision involves much more than "seeing" things. It includes our ability to see, recognize, and process information our eyes take in. Our visual system needs to decipher whether something is moving, judge its color, or even if we have seen the item in the past. In the same manner, our ears receive sound information in various pitches. It's from how we process sound waves that we form meaning from what we hear. Our nose is the receptor for scent information. Humans rely on scent as an extremely powerful sense since its receptors are directly related to our memory and the emotions associated with the scent. What goes into our mouths is deciphered by many receptors which pick up flavors and, equally important, humans learn to soothe themselves as babies when they place items into their mouths. We need to remember that our body forms associations with our sensations in order to help us to protect ourselves from danger and even to remember pleasurable events and repeat them later. So, our body requires information from other body systems in order to fully understand the world around us.

There are some additional senses that are lesser known. They are: proprioception; vestibular; and tactile. Let's discuss these lesser-known senses.

Proprioception involves receptors in our joints, tendons, and muscles. The receptors provide information on body position, movement, and stretch. Proprioceptive information gives us clues about body awareness. Close your eyes and stretch your arms above your head. Even with your eyes closed, you can "feel," or sense the position of your arms.

Vestibular information comes from receptors in our inner ear. Deep in the ear exist three semicircular canals filled with fluid. As the fluid moves, our receptors determine the position of our body in space. Gravity pulls on our bodies, and to remain upright our body is constantly trying to determine its position space. We gain an understanding of the importance of the vestibular system when we catch a cold and feel woozy or dizzy.

Tactile information originates from receptors in the skin. Our hands, feet, mouth, and skin exist to protect us, and via our tactile system give us information about the physical properties of an item, such as its texture, shape, temperature, and so on, as we explore it. Additionally, information about light or deep pressure touch comes from tactile receptors. We can determine if there is something heavy or something light touching our skin.

One of the most important points to remember is that the senses develop together and depend on the proper function of each other in order for our body to function best. When the ear becomes infected, the vestibular system is "off" since it is directly affected by the smooth flow of fluid in the inner ear. Illness, stress, injury, environmental, and internal factors all affect our sensory system in different ways.

Sensory and movement information bombard us as we move throughout our day. Receptors strategically placed in our bodies take in information. We process that information and form responses. So, we need to modulate and adapt to the challenges we face. Let's compare our body to a computer. The computer takes in information and compares it with pre-programmed sets of data. Based on the information the computer has, it responds and produces an output. So, when you type in the letter Z on the keyboard, the computer forms the letter Z on the screen. Of course, our body is quite a bit more complex than a computer as we experience emotions. Additionally, everyone's body is programmed differently based on biology and experiences so all or our letter Zs will appear differently.

Remember that everyone exists in a different level of sensory "alertness." For example, the radio in the business office is set at a volume of eight. Some of the staff feels the music is too loud for optimal concentration. They cannot work efficiently and are less productive as a result. Others disagree and state that the music should be louder. One of the staff members has slept poorly the night before and wishes the music was turned off so he can focus. However, the boss prefers the radio at the current level. The takeaway: We all experience events differently based on our body's programs, past experiences, and current emotions.

Learning is based on our experiences. As we interact with our world, we form positive and negative associations. Successful interactions produce pleasant memories and we show the desire to repeat them. With each success comes confidence. As a result, we form positive associations with a sensation or activity. However, we remember negative experiences and learn what *not* to do when something is unpleasant. Throughout our lives, our experiences and memories help shape our behaviors in order to keep us safe. If we touch a hot burner, we quickly learn not to repeat that behavior. Survival is our basic instinct.

Sensory processing should be a smooth and seamless process. When our bodies have difficulty processing information they receive, SPD may be the underlying issue. Imagine you are sitting in your back yard. Feel the cool breeze brushing lightly on your skin and the warm sunshine beating down on you. It's a great feeling to most of us! To those who experience SPD, simply sitting in the yard may be overwhelming. Let's imagine again: You are sitting in your yard and you feel the warmth of the sun, the cool breeze, the noise of the neighbor cutting grass, the smell of the sun lotion, the feel of the chair on your body, the tightness of your swimsuit, the tag on the garment, the sweat on your body; your eyes squint tightly due to the brightness of the sun, a bee buzzes by, you feel thirsty, the neighborhood children are yelling, the dog is barking. You cannot relax and read your book since you feel, see, and hear many different things. It's intense and stressful and quite overwhelming. Individuals with SPD often experience difficulty accommodating, or getting used to, sights, sounds, touch, pressure, tastes, and movement around them. As a result, they can become quite overwhelmed and upset quickly. Focusing on the task at hand becomes impossible and a meltdown may occur. Adults and children with decreased verbal skills often act out in frustration when they feel overstimulated. Their behavior speaks volumes about what their body feels. We must learn to be a detective in order to determine the "Why?" of the behavior. Why is she crying? Why is my child curled up in a ball? Why do I feel so upset?

Efficient sensory processing makes the difference between living comfortably and experiencing difficulty integrating the various sensations experienced throughout the day. When an illness or disability is present, the sensory system is often affected. Additionally, sensory processing disorders occur comorbidly (along with) with many other conditions. It's also important to remember that many typically developing children and many adults without other disabilities experience deficits in their sensory processing. So, sensory processing disorder can occur without any other medical or mental health disorder.

Oddly enough and to the great dismay of those who personally live with it, SPD is not an "official" diagnosis. As of the publication of this book, there is *no* official diagnosis of SPD. There has been a great deal of research by many dedicated individuals on the disorder as well as the integration of the sensory system. The American

Psychiatric Association is responsible for the publication entitled *Diagnostic and Statistical Manual of Mental Disorders* (DSM). The latest version of the manual is the DSM-5 and was released in May 2013. According to the American Psychiatric Association's website (American Psychiatric Association 2016):

> *Diagnostic and Statistical Manual of Mental Disorders, Fifth Edition (DSM-5)* is the standard classification of mental disorders used by mental health professionals in the United States. It is intended to be used in all clinical settings by clinicians of different theoretical orientations. It can be used by mental health and other health professionals, including psychiatrists and other physicians, psychologists, social workers, nurses, occupational and rehabilitation therapists, and counselors. *DSM-5* can also be used for research in clinical and community populations. It is also a necessary tool for collecting and communicating accurate public-health statistics.

Many researchers, such as those from the Sensory Processing Disorder Foundation, have dedicated their efforts to add SPD into the manual. It is important to note that sensory processing difficulty was added to the autism diagnostic information in the newest DSM. Remember (from earlier in this chapter) that Dr. A. Jean Ayres (an occupational therapist and educational psychologist) developed a theoretical framework and assessment for sensory integration. Today, occupational therapists continue to routinely document clients who present with functional limitations in daily life due to difficulties with sensory processing. Sensory processing difficulties occur in all ages and races, and in both males and females.

You Are Special

Believe it or not – there is no one else that is just like you. Your physical appearance, your voice and personality traits your habits, intelligence, personal tastes - all these make you one of a kind. Even your fingerprints distinguish you from every other human being - past, present, or future. You are not the product of some cosmic assembly line; you are unique. But the most important fact of your identity is that God created you in His own image (Genesis 1:27).

You are special indeed! God has total interest in you as an individual. The psalmist wrote in one of his most beautiful prayers, "I will praise Thee; for I am fearfully and wonderfully made." (Psalms 139:14). God knew you even before you were born. He had plans just for you, plans conceived in love. As you appreciate God's constant concern for you, you must begin to understand the awfulness of sin. He loves you so much; yet how often have you gone your own way?, turning your back on Him. Through sin, God's great design for your life is always blocked because His eyes cannot behold sin. But even in our sinful state, we are still precious to Him. He still sees us individuals with great value.

the psalmist declared, "How precious are Thy thoughts unto
how great is the sum of them! If I should count them, they are
umber than the sand" (Psalm 139:17-18). God is not an unfeeling,
rted monarch of the heavens. He feels our pains; He shares our
s. He cares, and He considers each one of us important enough to

t, He loves us so much that He gave His only Son to die for our sins.
rein is love," the Bible says, "not that we loved God but that He loved
and sent His Son to be the propitiation [full payment] for our sins"
John 4:10).
Because you are special to God, He wants to forgive you and give you a full,
meaningful life. When you trust in Jesus Christ and let Him put your life
together, the Bible says you become "God's masterpieces, created in
Christ Jesus" (Ephesians 2:10, paraphrase). Can anyone be more special
than that?

Yes, you are valuable to God! If you've never trusted Jesus Christ for
your salvation, you can pray the following prayer and be saved today:

*"Lord, thank You for sending Jesus Christ to die for my sins and rise from the
dead so that I can know Your forgiveness and live with You forever. Right
now I ask Jesus Christ to be my Saviour. so I can live as the special creation
that You intended. Thank you Lord for saving me, in Jesus name. Amen".*
Congratulations! You are now saved

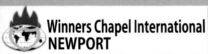

Winners Chapel International
NEWPORT

Ty Derwen, Church Road, Newport. NP19 7EJ
Sunday Service: 10:00 am
Wednesday Service: 6:30pm - 8:00pm
Tel: 07901024213 | 073988004433
E: newport@winners-chapel.org.uk

WINNERS' SATELLITE
FELLOWSHIP LOCATION

Both of the authors of this book, many of their family members and clients, and others experience difficulties with processing sensory information. It's extremely frustrating that we live with SPD every day and feel its effects, yet many professionals and some insurance companies have not yet officially recognized it. We encourage our readers to continue to research and fund studies that assist professionals in their attempts to add SPD into subsequent diagnostic manuals. Occupational therapists around the world are working diligently to study and describe it.

What problems result from SPD?

There are other ways OTs look at sensory processing. Our body requires information gained from the senses in order to regulate our posture, position in space, and gross and fine motor coordination. According to research by Bundy *et al.* (2007), our sensory system is responsible for so much more than just taking in and making sense of our surroundings. The information received is processed and used to make adjustments in our body which affect functioning in daily life. For example, if I'm not receiving *or* correctly processing information about gravity from my vestibular system, I may not be able to hold my body upright when I'm sitting at my desk. Fatigue, postural problems, and the appearance of being "lazy" may result. It's easy to see how quickly a student can be labeled due to something well beyond his control! Another example: If I cannot feel my pencil due to deficits in my tactile system or its processing, I may not be able to hold it properly to form letters. The plan my body creates is inefficient as a result of my sensory processing deficits. The term *dyspraxia* means difficulty creating and performing coordinated movement patterns. In our case, as a result of the incorrect processing of sensory information, someone may have difficulty planning what they want their bodies to do. Can you imagine how frustrating this might be? All areas of the body systems may be affected: vision, hearing, motion, touch, movement, even our internal organs need to process information to make subconscious decisions using sensory information.

We must point out that many individuals with SPD have no other illness, injury, or disability. However, SPD often occurs in combination with other conditions. We call this a comorbid condition. When someone has inefficient sensory processing or SPD, many difficulties in daily life may result. Remember that our sensory system is designed to protect us. If a client experiences an overwhelmed sensory system or becomes stressed, hormones are released which cause a fight-or-flight reaction. It is during a stress response that a person may act out with physical or verbal aggression. When someone is fearful for their own safety, it's natural to escape the situation and complete whatever is necessary to gain a feeling of safety again.

Oftentimes in children and adults who experience inefficient sensory processing, behavior difficulties occur. This is especially true when rudimentary verbal skills are lacking. If someone cannot describe her fear in words, she may exercise aggression in attempt to gain control of what's happening to her. So, when we regulate the sensory system, the person generally feels more in control of their body and can learn other skills which require focus and concentration. In essence, the sensory processing system is a "basic" system that should be balanced (regulated) so that higher learning and functioning may occur.

Sensory processing disorder can negatively affect and limit daily living, school, and work activities due to the barrage of sensory information coming into the brain. For adults at work, it can be nearly impossible to work in a noisy environment, such as an office setting with cubicles. The noise of phones ringing, people talking, people walking by, and office machinery noise can make it difficult or nearly impossible for person with SPD to perform their job. People adapt by choosing jobs where the sensory input is minimal; as a result, they can often be underemployed.

Likewise, children in school may outwardly display their SPD responses by behaving badly or having meltdowns into screaming or hitting because they do not yet have the coping skills. Adults will avoid or walk away from an overly sensory situation, but children do not have that option. Often these children will be moved to small classes in special education rooms due to their behavior.

Occupational therapists should continue to work on developing concrete and evidence-based outcome measures for those with sensory processing difficulties (Schaaf *et al.* 2014). However, for those living with SPD, there is no question that life with SPD can be difficult. For either an adult or child, SPD can negatively affect daily living. They will avoid sensory-rich situations, such as going to a fair, a museum, or an amusement park, limiting their pleasurable activities. Necessary life tasks, such as going to the bank, grocery shopping, or errands, can be difficult. Adults will often alter when they do an activity, such as going grocery shopping, to very early in the morning when there are few people in the store. For some, driving can be difficult because of the need to pay attention to so much movement and noise at once. Some people may have to narrow down what they can wear due to clothing tags, tight waists, or the seams in socks which can feel irritating or even painful.

Generally, a person with sensory processing disorder seeks sensory input, avoids sensory input, or can seek or avoid in different sensory areas. There is no "right" way to have sensory processing disorder and the functional deficits resulting vary greatly from person to person.

Weighted blankets, then, attempt to increase overall body regulation by providing input to pressure receptors in the tactile system. Often combined with other sensory items, blankets are a part of important therapeutic techniques. The goal is that when the person's body is better regulated, they may feel more calm and safe, and move to other activities.

Exploring deep pressure

Many people have said to me that a weighted blanket feels like a hug, which makes them feel relaxed, calm, and less anxious. Studies on touch show that it is essential to the physical growth of children, and for adults it can lower stress and make them emotionally and physically healthier.

As an autistic child, I did not like being touched, and I still don't like it sometimes. I live in Minnesota, and we're a huggy bunch, so I have had to get used to it. I also now like hugging my loved ones, but touch from strangers, such as a touch on my arm or handshakes, can feel invasive.

Research has shown that hugs release oxytocin (National Institutes of Health 2007). This hormone is known to act on the limbic system (the parts of the brain that are concerned with emotion and motivation) in the brain. When oxytocin is released, humans experience decreased anxiety, feelings of comfort and bonding, and decreasing stress. Additionally, hugs release dopamine. Magnetic resonance imaging (MRI) scans completed by several scientists have revealed that the brain releases dopamine when humans are hugged or even when they anticipate a hug. For a discussion of the link between hugging and the release of dopamine see University of Miami School of Medicine Touch Research

Institute (2013). Any time pleasure hormones are released, the body experiences physiological changes. Decreased blood pressure, decreases in heart rate, and increased ability to fight infections have been studied and proven to be associated with deep pressure and hug stimulation (Edelson *et al.* 1999).

Fantastically, hugs have a therapeutic effect on the body and brain. Relaxation, feelings of safety, and security are free to those who are able to hug another person.

Interestingly, there is a product on the market called an "internet pajama" (Teh *et al.* n.d.). The wearer can feel a hug from a person at a distance through the internet. The sender hugs a doll that can sense varying levels of pressure. It sends these signals to the jacket that produces the pressure on the wearer. Air pockets produce the pressure, along with heating elements to produce warmth.

Massage

In studies at the University of Miami Touch Research Institute, researchers found that moderate pressure massage reduces stress hormones, lowers blood pressure, and slows heart rate. According to Tiffany Field, the director of the institute, moderate pressure massage also improves immune function. In one study, adults who received a chair massage performed better on math calculations after the massage.

Deep pressure massage relaxes by lowering stress hormones and may reduce inflammatory substances by increasing white blood cells, which help in fighting viruses or disease.

Our body is constantly working to achieve "regulation." This is a state in which we are able to derive the most meaning and learning from our environment. For example, when someone is excited to learn, has had a completely balanced meal, and feels at his best, he will most likely be in a more ready state to learn than someone who has not slept through the night, is hungry, and agitated. To achieve regulation, our body constantly receives information. The parasympathetic (rest and digest) and the sympathetic systems (fight or flight) are critical for our survival. Information about our environment is constantly scanned by the body's sensory system in order to determine if our safety is in jeopardy. The sympathetic system activates the fight-or-flight response and excites the body, whereas the parasympathetic system works to relax the body and get it back to its resting (or regulated) state. When we determine a situation is "dangerous," our body releases cortisol, among other stress hormones. In contrast, relaxation and massage, or stimulation to our tactile system, usually activate the parasympathetic system. However, since everyone's perception of touch is different based on our body's system and past experiences, the amount of pressure used in massage is subjective.

Stacie Piehowski from Kalla Lily Salon and Spa in Maple Grove, Minnesota, says: "The concept of the gliding/kneading techniques is to get circulation going and relax the client; compression would relate to the weighted blanket effect, to just compress and give a larger surface area pressure versus just a pinpointed area."

Oftentimes in therapeutic settings and in massage clinics, clients with conditions such as fibromyalgia have difficulty tolerating deep pressure. On the other hand, clients with autism or multiple sclerosis, or those who have higher sensory thresholds (or require more input in order to register sensory stimuli) may prefer a deeper touch/pressure massage. Stacie suspects, and our research of the current literature and principles of sensory and massage technique leads us to believe, that massage and weighted blankets may both engage the compression, stretch, and traction receptors in the body. In massage, compression is activated by pressing into the body with open hands and covering as much surface area as possible with a firm pressure. Occupational and physical therapists, among others, utilize massage as a regular treatment modality.

As we complete our daily routine we tend to live "in our own head" as we consider our busy schedules, stressors of life, work, and so on. We often forget that our bodies require tender care. It's not until our body becomes injured or "screams" for attention that we realize how much we neglect our body's needs. A common example is when a body develops a condition such as carpal tunnel syndrome or plantar fasciitis due to repetitive overuse. We are learning more and more about the mind–body effect and how mindfulness techniques, such as meditation or biofeedback, affect the body. The brain and body are commonly thought of as separate entities, but knowledge is growing as we learn more about the mind–body connection. Some of it has entered the mainstream through articles in health magazines about how exercise can make you happy because it releases feel-good endorphins in the brain. Endorphins work on the receptors in your brain that reduce the feeling of pain. This "runner's high" triggers the positive feelings that are similar to that of morphine. Hence, vigorous exercise is recommended for people who are dealing with depression.

While some concepts show how the body affects the mind as is the case with massage or exercise, more study is needed to learn more about how a deep pressure on the body affects the mind.

Neuroscience

I interviewed neuroscientist and author Gary Wenk, professor at Ohio State University, who talked about the mind–body effect from the point of view of the body affecting the mind.

With weighted blankets he reminded me that we do not have to know why it works, just that it does:

> When I teach this course to undergraduates, I always remind them that when we talk about antidepressants or any antipsychotics, the FDA [Food and Drug Administration] doesn't require that we understand how anything works, only that it's effective and safe.
>
> From my standpoint as a neuroscientist, I would have predicted that if an autistic child felt better in your blanket then so would a person with schizophrenia and so would a person with dementia, because there's a lot of overlap. Given the similarities we are beginning to see, a whole spectrum of disorders have connections. Researchers who are doing scanning with fMRI (functional magnetic resonance imaging, a technique that measures brain activity) are finding that there are some interesting links that underlie biological connections that we never thought existed.

Wenk describes how the sensory system works. A mosquito bite can be painful or itchy, and you find that if you scratch all around it, even if you don't scratch on it, the itch goes away. Not all sensory input is entirely represented in your brain, so the body's solution is simply to have a bit of overlap: by scratching on the area right next to the mosquito bite, you can actually overwhelm the sensory input from the mosquito bite. A little bit of sensory input comes from your scratching around the bite, and a little bit comes in from the irritation of the mosquito bite, and they reach a point in the spinal column where it chooses which signals it lets through, the itch or scratch around it. If you scratch a lot, you overwhelm the itch's signal, so the scratch wins by getting its signal through to the brain. After a few moments, the scratch wanes, and the mosquito bite wins:

> Given this, it might be seen as an advantage, and it could be seen as a disadvantage in how our nervous system works, so that sometimes doing odd sensory things does make us feel better. But let me make a completely separate point and then pull these two things together.
>
> A lot of my students are on are on SSRIs (selective serotonin reuptake inhibitors—a class of antidepressants). It's hard to believe that people in their teens and twenties can be on SSRIs, but I think my class attracts them. They always want to know, "Why am I depressed and why does this drug help me? What's it doing?" So this is kind of analogous to what you often hear from the patients and families who use weighted blankets: "Why does this make me feel better?"
>
> Now, if you look at the web for SSRIs and even just look at their name, you're going to get the impression that blocking the reuptake of serotonin must be the reason that I feel better. After all, that's what the drugs are called. And when they were first designed, that's what they did, and they do help people. And when it comes to the brain and chemistry it's never that simple.
>
> Let's say that you're a depressed person and you took your SSRI. Within half an hour, I can guarantee that you're having serotonin released in your brain. Yet, you don't feel this lack of depression, and you're still depressed. Weeks go by, maybe a month, maybe two, and then finally you notice "I don't feel as depressed anymore." There is a massive time disconnect between when the drugs are producing serotonin and when you

feel better. So when you answer the question "Why do I feel better, was it due to serotonin?," the answer ends up being no, not really. I know that one thing we discovered is that just because the drug can do something, and I know what it does in your brain, that is not the reason it actually helps you. The fact that you take a blanket and lay it on somebody and they feel comforted is real, but the explanation may not be known.

So the question becomes, What does that part of your brain do? Let me give you an explanation.

If you are sitting next to someone you really really like, and they start petting your arm—let's say in the direction that the hair on your skin lies down. And they are just petting you because they like you, just a gentle "I really care for you" petting. If someone asked you "Does that feel nice?" you would say "Yes."

Now let's remove that nice person and put in someone who is creepy. When that person does the same movement on the same arm you would become frightened. It would feel uncomfortable and you would want to run away screaming.

There is a part of the brain that decides if you like a particular touch, and that part of the brain is called the insula. All of the sensory information that comes into the brain, like light touch, deep touch, and so on, needs to be put together somewhere, so there is a part of the brain that seems to respond and says is this painful, is this pleasurable, do you like it, not like it?—the insula would be the part of your cortex that processes that. There are parts that process the painful things, and there is a part that processes the taste of chocolate when you really like it and when you eat too much chocolate and don't like it anymore, there is a part of that same region of the cortex that processes that as well.

Knowing these few things, what the fMRI people at Stanford have done, they have started asking the question, since the insula is involved in sensory processing and if these kids with autism have a problem with sensory processing, let's take a look at their brains when we are touching them.

What they found is that the insula does not work as well. It does not respond as well, it is thinner when you look at the anatomy, it does not seem to be wired up properly in certain groups of people—the ones who have sensory disorders, those who have chronic pain, and in autistic children.

They are now taking people with specific disorders, say schizophrenic, autistic, or so on, and putting them in a scanner—this scanning has gotten cheap enough now that you can do this with hundreds of people.

So the question becomes where can we point to in the brain? This goes back almost a hundred years or more where they would measure bumps on the skull; now they are looking at light and dark areas of activity within these individuals.

The proprioceptive senses are not just a one-way street that we get information on: We also modify back to our sensory inputs to sort of alter what we experience. A good example of this is the sense of taste. When you first start eating something and you are hungry, we know that the taste buds are far more active than when you are not hungry anymore—that is your brain telling your taste buds to stop responding to everything as if it is so wonderful. The same things actually happen to all of our sensory systems.

So the question becomes where is this multisensory experience produced by the blanket actually happening? If you imagine you are an autistic person and your nervous system is being bombarded by something sensory and your brain is trying to combat it by sending signals back out saying, "Stop it, stop it"—you have this horrible sensory loop where you cannot get things to calm down. One of the ways to combat this is to, in a way, "itch your brain." Like in the scratching example I spoke of earlier, by sending other signals (such as hand waving) it overcomes the "itching" sensations and works to calm the brain down.

If you now imagine your whole body is covered by itchiness and I took something abrasive or containing menthol and rubbed it all over you, you would feel better—it would overwhelm the itchy sensations with other sensations. This is the same as over-the-counter pain/itching treatments. Many of these contain menthol, which produces a broad sensory stimulation which overwhelms the pain sensors coming in.

The weighted blanket is doing the same thing with broad pressure all over the skin. You are taking advantage of how the sensory system is wired; you are producing large sensory inputs causing the calming effect in the brain. Now, are dopamine or serotonin released? Maybe, but I have no way of knowing. There are scientists who will make the claim that there is serotonin released but this is not really based on fact—no one can be sure. If someone wants to use this or believe this, that is fine. That kind of goes to the FDA's philosophy that it does not matter *how* it works, as long it *does* work.

There would be all kinds of caveats that you would have to throw in when describing how your weighted blankets work that would make it a very complex story. You could spin a story involving all forms of chemicals in the brain, but no one knows for sure what inputs cause which chemicals to be released.

We do know the insula is involved and that it does become active with touch, but also the insula is involved with other sensory inputs as well. Such as if you are placed in a scanner and listen to some music you like, there will be activity detected in the insula. But by the same token if it is music you don't like, the insula will also show activity. This is the part of the brain that judges sensory inputs (light, touch, sound, and so on) and tells you if you like them or not.

But again I will say, it really does not matter how it works: it is only important that it makes them feel better.

Chapter 4

Professional Settings

Occupational therapy

What is occupational therapy?

The profession of occupational therapy has existed since the 1700s. During the Age of Enlightenment, people sought answers and took a new look at old ideas. Many people lived with mental illness and were treated horribly. People began to realise that instead of banning those with mental illness from society, they might be helped by exercise, through completing activities involving their own interests, and considering stresses in their daily lives. Later, in the 1800s, crafts were added as therapeutic activities. Eventually, in the early 1900s, a nurse, Susan E. Tracy, realized the importance of using her patient's interests to improve their functional outcomes. She wrote a book about bringing crafts to those who had mental illness. The profession of occupational therapy then "officially" began! Today, occupational therapists work in many settings, including mental health, hospitals, rehabilitation, pediatrics, geriatrics, home health care, and many more.

The official definition according to the World Federation of Occupational Therapists (2011):

Occupational therapy is a client-centred health profession concerned with promoting health and well being through occupation. The primary goal of occupational therapy is to enable people to participate in the activities of everyday life. Occupational therapists achieve this outcome by working with people and communities to enhance their ability to engage in the occupations they want to, need to, or are expected to do, or by modifying the occupation or the environment to better support their occupational engagement.

Occupational therapists assist people to function independently during activities of daily living (ADLs). The training OTs receive includes anatomy, psychology, human development, philosophy, neuroanatomy, chemistry, biology, kinesiology, sensory systems, and activity adaptation. The varied training allows OTs to determine how a specific illness or disability affects the entire person and his daily life. They look at the "whole person" instead of the brain or the arm or the muscles. Additionally, therapists receive on-the-job training for two periods of 12 weeks in their specialty area. This allows OTs to focus on and become experienced in the specific area or age group of clients they will be working with. One of the most important things OTs do is to adapt the client's environment. For example, if a client experiences a meltdown (stress reaction), the therapist creates a "cool down" area. The area may include weighted blankets, relaxing music, cards with breathing exercises to slow down breaths, or low lighting. Further, education of the caregiver is one of the primary jobs of the therapist. Teaching ways to increase function, involving the caregiver in therapy sessions, and providing home therapy programs are common strategies OTs use.

An important way therapists impact lives is by training clients on future wellness and prevention of future disease or disability. For example, OTs routinely recommend products specially designed to improve function. Adaptive plates, specialized bathroom equipment, and products for improving sensory integration are recommended. Children who require help with daily life tasks may use fidget toys, weighted blankets and other garments, special chairs, and tools to decrease chewing on inappropriate items.

Weighted blankets are one of the items commonly recommended for children through people of all ages. Instructing the client and the caregiver on the use and safety of the equipment remains one of the most important tasks to ensure proper use. Purchase options are discussed. In fact, there are entire catalogues and businesses that publish catalogues for those with special needs, illness, and injuries.

How are weighted blankets used at an OT clinic?

Occupational therapy clinics in all settings employ weighted blankets to assist clients in the process of self-regulation. According to Champagne *et al.* (2015), weighted blankets "are a class of sensory processing-related interventions that utilize deep pressure touch stimulation (DPTS)." Oftentimes, they are used when a patient feels out of balance and disorganized emotionally or physically. The blanket is always optional and provides a feeling of comfort similar to a hug. When someone is hugged, the chemical oxytocin may be released. Oxytocin affects receptors in our bodies that correspond with pleasure. Although there is no current proof that weighted blankets themselves cause the body to release oxytocin, for most of us it feels great to receive a hug from others and the blanket is often described as feeling "like a hug."

Therapists sometimes use a fabric tube made of stretchable Lycra fibers to emulate deep pressure. However, the weight of the blanket may stimulate the deep pressure or touch receptors of the tactile system as well as providing a more uniform pressure. It's suggested that the blanket use is coupled with deep breathing, relaxation techniques, visualizations, or other calming activities.

A special area of the therapy room, clinic, school, or hospital may be set up as a sensory room. This generally includes a weighted blanket as an option for self-calming. Additionally, the weighted blanket is often used as part of a grounding technique. According to leading professor of psychiatry Dr. Lisa Najavitis, a grounding technique is used to balance someone between feeling too much and too little (Najavitis 2002). Grounding helps to keep us in the present (here and now) and assists us in mind and body connections. It may be that the weight of the blanket provides the physical input to the body. The blanket may be used either while seated or when lying down. One of the biggest benefits is that a child or adult should be able to both apply and remove the blanket. The feeling of being in control is quite important and therapeutic for so many people.

How does OT work for SPD?

Some occupational therapists choose to work in the area of sensory integration. Sensory integration is one of the frameworks used by OTs. It's important that the distinction is made: These OTs are not "sensory integration therapists" but are occupational therapists who use sensory techniques. When a client comes for an assessment, the OT chooses assessments related to SPD, looks at how sensory issues affect the daily life of the client, and makes a treatment plan which includes goals agreed upon by the team. OTs who work in sensory integration receive training by other therapists with SPD experience. Additionally, there are many courses in sensory integration and sensory processing disorders. Continuing education is a requirement for all therapists to maintain their certification and licensing.

Therapists utilize sensory integrative techniques with clear goals to improve function. Occupational therapists provide sensory and movement opportunities that challenge the client over time. Interventions are client-driven and as each challenge is successfully completed, the client builds his confidence level along with his competence in completing the task. Additionally, the OT can assist in modifying the client's environment for success. Therapists often collect data to determine the effectiveness of interventions for the client since the best way to validate something is to continue to document effectiveness with data and research.

The tools OTs use when working with clients who have SPD include swings, brushes, weighted blankets, spinning boards, large exercise balls, vibrating pillows, putty, and elastic exercise bands. The techniques OTs use can be employed by all ages and populations. When children have difficulty knowing where their bodies are in relation to the space they are in, the therapist may choose to use a brush on the child's skin to stimulate the receptors in the "tactile" areas. Also, the child may be asked to swing or bounce on a large ball. Oftentimes, the OT asks the child to lie on a mat and uses massage or rolls a ball gently on his back. They may play "sandwich" by placing a weighted blanket (pretend meat or cheese) on the child (pretending to be the bun). Silly condiments are often added with vibration being the ketchup or mayo. Sensory therapy is designed to be fun and enjoyable. *Most* importantly, the client must remain in control of the therapeutic interventions. He/ she may request to stop if a therapeutic technique is at all uncomfortable.

The question is often asked, "How long does it take for the effects of sensory-based therapy interventions (such as the application of a weighted blanket) to work?" It's impossible to provide a concrete answer as some feel the effects immediately and others require many sessions until the intervention that fits the person's unique needs is determined. It is known that when a therapist applies vestibular interventions (spinning, swinging, head upside-down), the effects can last from six to eight hours. The effects of proprioceptive interventions last from two to four hours.

Each person's sensory system is vastly different. Remember that when our body perceives sensory information, our brains make sense of them by comparing to past experiences. One of the most important jobs of our sensory systems is to protect us from danger. We move from a state of rest to a panic response when we smell smoke, hear a fire alarm, see flames, feel intense heat, experience pain, and so on. When sensory processing is not functioning optimally, some individuals "feel" or perceive too much or too little.

What is the impact when the sensory system is wired incorrectly? Many people with SPD avoid preferred activities (activities other people usually enjoy) such as talking in a coffee shop with a friend, being able to go out for an evening, or being able to have the windows open in the summer due to the "assault" of noise. Sensory processing disorder includes the level of alertness in which our body exists. Additionally, SPD may limit ability to work. "I haven't the balance to be a waitress. I can't think in a cubicle with noise surrounding me. I would get quickly confused in a fast food restaurant with all the movement, smells, and sounds." Occupational therapists can quickly determine if someone is aware of and has difficulty filtering out sensory information that is not relevant or useful. If the receptors exist in a heightened state, every sight, sound, touch, smell, movement is processed at the same level, thus causing an extreme overstress of the body as it attempts to respond.

In contrast, some people's bodies do not receive and/or process important information. This can sometimes result in danger, such as decreased awareness of injury. A patient may report, "My husband will say, 'How did you get that bruise?' I run into things and I have falls, some of which have caused injury beyond a bruise." Oftentimes, children with decreased (hypo-responsivity) experience throw themselves from higher playground equipment or crash and bump into objects or people intentionally in an attempt to "feel" their body in space.

One of the most important takeaway points is that SPD can cause different parts of our bodies to perceive information in different ways. This is also true in clients with illness and injury, or mental health conditions such as PTSD. For example, a patient may report that all noises sound intense but senses of taste and smell are decreased. Another person may feel touch (even light touch) as painful, but balance is decreased due to vestibular receptors having difficulty responding to movement and gravity. This mixed hypo- and hyper-sensory processing is common and the OT assists clients through various assessments, activities, and observation. A unique and individualized treatment plan is formed. Each specific client's interests are considered and the impact of SPD on their daily life is determined.

Hospital use

Treatment for mental health remains a top priority in today's health care. Mental health disorders are vast and varied. Some patients benefit from visiting a therapist on a regular basis in an office or clinic setting. Recommendations are made and a home program is followed. Often, medication is coupled with behavior or cognitive therapy. When a more intensive program is deemed necessary, there may be an inpatient stay. Weighted blanket use in hospital inpatient mental health facilities is on the rise.

Restraint reduction

Today's mental health facilities and inpatient units differ greatly from those of the past. Thankfully, we continue to evolve and change to improve the environment and support for those who struggle with a mental illness. One of the main differences is the restrictions on the use of restraints, including chains, straps, tying with sheets, and other methods which were commonly employed in the past with no regard for the physical or mental damage caused. Restraint is defined as:

> any method, drug or medication, physical or mechanical device, material or equipment, that immobilizes or reduces the ability of an individual to move any part of the body freely, particularly when used to restrict or manage a client's behavior or movement. (U.S. Department of Health and Human Services 2006)

In April 2002, President George W. Bush created the New Freedom Commission on Mental Health. The goal was to "study mental health delivery systems, and to make recommendations that would enable adults with serious mental illness and children with serious emotional disturbances to live, work, learn, and participate fully in their communities." Results showed that changes were needed, and the report outlined six goals, including that mental health services be consumer-driven and educating the public that mental health impacts overall health.

Since a major area of concern included restraint reduction, new focus areas include the use of sensory and comfort rooms. Weighted blankets can be used as a replacement therapy, since it helps patients feel calmer, thus reducing the need for restraint and seclusion. Occupational therapists are specifically trained to evaluate how disease and mental health concerns affect the entire person. The cognitive, emotional, and physical aspects are considered when formulating a treatment plan. The increases in understanding of sensory processing disorder and the impact that sensory integration has on function are adding to the use of alternative and patient driven techniques.

In an interview, Clarissa Mireau of St. Joseph's Hospital, St. Paul, Minnesota described how the use of OT has grown in the hospital setting. It is common for weighted blankets to be used in pediatric settings for sensory issues, and their use in the adult population is increasing. They are now used as an anxiety-reducing and grounding technique. Weighted blanket benefits encompass people with a history of trauma, borderline personality disorder (BPD), and self-injurious behaviors. Mireau reported that:

> there seems to be a connection between trauma and seeking sensory behavior so patients seek sensory input. For example, on a locked unit there are close spaces which can be anxiety producing. One particular patient would sit on the edge of the group or not come at all, or she became upset when any chaos existed on the unit. We used a weighted blanket wrapped round her tightly and she was able to participate, and it increased her comfort level and improved her follow through.

The staff at St. Joseph's Hospital utilize a well-rounded treatment team including OT, spirituality, chemical dependency education, behavioral therapy, and small groups. Some groups focus on sobriety and use of illegal substances. All patients participate in a primary group with a licensed chemical dependency counselor. Patient involvement in treatment options remains of critical importance.

Each patient's needs are considered by the team. Anxiety can be a big issue for many of the patients in hospital settings and obtaining patient input about environmental concerns helps to lessen worry and stress. Many adults do not have awareness of sensory processing disorder, and when patients understand their own sensory needs, they are better able to manage their need to either seek or avoid various sensory stimuli.

After Mireau completes sensory profiles on the clients, she is able to ask the doctor to write an order to get insurance coverage for a blanket.

Another way St. Joseph's helps patients deal with some of the challenges that arise while on the unit is by using a weighted blanket. They have found that some patients who use weighted blankets find them very effective for getting them "over the hump" during withdrawing or detoxing as this is a shock to their system.

The staff have been blown away by how helpful a weighted blanket is. Oftentimes, the use of weighted blankets offers a great way to help patients and the entire treatment team with sensory processing issues. They are hopeful that the use of the blankets may eventually decrease some patients' chemical dependency as many of their patients have a dual diagnosis. When one patient sees another using the blanket, they often request one.

Gretchen Prohofsky, OTR/L BH, Allied Health Manager at Regions Hospital, St. Paul, Minnesota, writes:

> Many individuals with mental health disturbances also have a co-occurring sensory processing disorder. Since we began using weighted blankets on our inpatient mental health units, we have seen a drastic decline in the use of seclusion and restraint, as well as safety sitters.

Some of the common themes we hear from patients are that they feel calmer, more grounded, safe and secure, centered, improved concentration, decreased stress and anxiety, as well as having improved sleep. (personal communication, 2014)

She says the patients are very interested in learning about their sensory processing disorder and request reading materials to increase their understanding. The patients are also receptive to utilizing additional sensory tools to positively impact their quality of life.

According to a 2007 American Occupational Therapy Association presentation by Champagne, Mullen, and Dickinson titled *Exploring the Safety and Effectiveness of the Use of Weighted Blankets with Adult Populations*, 63 percent of study participants rated lower anxiety on survey called the State Trait Anxiety Index (STAI-10) with the use of a 30-pound blanket; 78 percent reported that the use of a 30-pound weighted blanket helped to reduce perceived level of anxiety. Of importance is this study's use of physiological measures—pulse rate and blood pressure— to determine key outcomes. Guidelines were utilized which reflected common physiological signs of anxiety. Champagne *et al.* 2007 reported:

Any readings that were outside the safe range were outside of that range prior to the use of the WB, demonstrating that the weighted blanket was not the cause of pulse and blood pressure readings falling outside of the safe ranges.

Therefore, results showed that all 20 participants' vital sign measurements (blood pressure, pulse oximetry (oxygen saturation in the blood), and pulse rate) stayed within the safe range.

The latest study (Champagne *et al.* 2015) investigated the effects of the use of a 30-pound weighted blanket measured by pulse rate, pulse oximetry, blood pressure, and self-report, among others.

The study was completed in an inpatient mental health institution. Thirty-pound blankets with both a fleece or cotton fabric side were utilized. Only the fleece side was placed against the patient. Two sessions occurred, one (control) without the blanket and one (experimental) with the blanket. Vital signs of patients ensured safety when using the blankets while lying down. Each session lasted for five minutes. The results of the study concluded that the use of the weighted blanket was safe for 100 percent of the participants based on measurements of vital signs and effective for 60 percent in reducing self-rated anxiety on the STAI-10.

While completing research for this book, we found only two published studies specifically on weighted blankets. Most of the "standard" wearing schedules are based on studies of weighted vests, hats, or other wearable products. Since very few studies have been published about weighted blankets, we urge other professionals using them to consider undertaking further research.

Weighted blankets have been shown to benefit other populations as well. Surgeries, illness, and injury can cause great anxiety and disruption of a patient's sensory system. The calming and regulating effects of the blankets carries over to patients in all treatment areas.

Some considerations for use are the same as with any medical equipment. The fabric of weighted blankets for use in hospitals must be able to be cleaned. Also, the use of a weighted blanket must be monitored if the patient has signs of infection, wounds, circulatory deficits, or diabetes, among other conditions. Patients and caregivers must be taught to monitor their skin integrity, temperature, respiratory rate, and/or blood pressure. Weighted blankets should be considered as a medical treatment and not just a "feel-good" application. This is especially true when the blankets are recommended for home use upon discharge from the hospital.

Actual use in a hospital setting

Each hospital sets its own rules concerning the use of blankets. Of utmost concern is the safety of the patients. Oftentimes, patients are admitted due to suicidal thoughts or actions. It is critical to remove all items which could be used in attempt to self-harm. Items include shoelaces, cords, and drawstrings. Strict rules for staff and visitors must be followed to ensure the safety of everyone. Doors to inpatient units are often locked in order to prevent escape during a severe episode of psychosis. Hospitals seek safe and effective ways of calming patients and reducing anxiety. Some hospitals utilize weighted neck wraps; however, if a patient becomes agitated or hostile during an exacerbation they may be used as a weapon.

Infection control is important for preventing the spread of infectious disease. Hospitals need to learn specifications about cleaning and fabric care from the weighted blanket company.

Here are some basic questions about infection control:

- How do you clean them?

- Can they be wiped down with germicide?

- Do you have documentation from the fabric mill (maker) on what types of cleaners can and cannot be used on the fabric? For example, the fabric I used could not be cleaned with bleach. Keep in mind that the fabric company may not test every cleaner on the market, or they may have not tested the newest cleaners.

- What properties does the fabric have, such as the feel, warmth, stretch, and other properties? To prevent ulcerations, a fabric must be "breathable," such as cotton. Ask for a fabric sample.

- Can they be washed in high-temperature (>160°F) hospital laundries, or do they have to be cleaned in a "home" machine on the unit?

When using weighted blankets, make sure to follow these guidelines:

- The patient must be able to remove the blanket by peeling it back.

- Staff must use proper lifting techniques.

- If the patient is lying down, place the blanket on the patient's shins and pull the blanket up to the shoulders, then pull it over the patient's feet.

- Hospital staff have told me that patients can be disoriented and panicky after surgery, so the blanket helps to calm them down. If they are used for post-surgery, follow doctor's orders on whether the blanket can cover the patient's entire body. If it can't, place the blanket on a part of the body that has not been operated on, again with the doctor's approval.

- If a patient has growing anxiety or other symptoms, use the blanket at the earliest sign of agitation to help bring the patient's anxiety level down before symptoms become extreme.

- Use smaller blankets, lap blankets, or shoulder wraps during group time.

- During psychotherapy sessions, use a smaller blanket. A therapist in Rock Hill, South Carolina said that it can help lower the client's anxiety level while working through issues such as trauma.

- If using duvet covers, have the end closed with Velcro toward the patient's feet so the rough edge does not irritate the patient's neck.

- Patients who self-harm could use the hook part of the Velcro on the duvet covers to harm themselves so use other safer methods of closing the duvet cover; use a duvet cover that doesn't close at one end, or don't use a duvet cover at all.

- Weighted blankets with plastic pellets as the filling can also be frozen, with the cooling effect lasting about 40 minutes. Do not use them as an alternative to other proven techniques for reducing fever.

Comfort/multisensory rooms

Inpatient hospitals desire to provide best practice for their patients. Sensory and comfort rooms are becoming more common. Studies have shown that patients are more compliant in treatment when they are involved in the planning of goals and activities. Independent skills blossom when patients are included as part of the treatment team. Additionally, when a hospital creates a sensory room, specific considerations are made. According to a study by Cummings, Grandfield, and Coldwell (2010), the use of sensory rooms and rooms in which patients are comfortable decreases the use of restraints. The study confirms ideas which support comfortable environments for patients.

Coupling calming colors and furniture with soothing music and lowered lighting evokes feelings of peace and comfort.

Sensory rooms are gaining new popularity as their benefits are reaching people everywhere. Generally, a sensory room is specifically designed to fit a person's specific sensory needs. The room is designed for exploration and is person-driven, meaning that the user is in charge of how they use the room. Sensory rooms are used in all settings and by individuals of all ages. In fact, nursing homes, skilled nursing facilities, mental health units, and schools often contain a sensory room. Some of the basic equipment found in a sensory space includes calm lighting (sometimes fiberoptic with slowly changing colors—*no* fluorescent lights); fidget toys; relaxing music or sounds such as waves, chimes, or white noise; bean bags, weighted blankets, soft cushions; and swings, rocking chairs, and other equipment to provide movement experiences. Sensory rooms can become quite expensive if the equipment is purchased from catalogues for special needs. There are many more economical design ideas to be found on Pinterest and other social media. The best sensory rooms are designed with a person's specific sensory needs in mind and with the help of an occupational therapist specifically trained in sensory processing disorders.

The uses for sensory rooms may vary. For example, when an individual experiences a period of frustration, aggression, and overall body and sensory dysregulation, he may go to a calming environment with the goal of calming in mind.

A Snoezelen room—from the Dutch verbs *snuffelen* (to explore) and *doezelen* (to relax)—is a specific room used for individuals with significant mental impairment. Two Dutch psychologists designed rooms which improved communication and encouraged clients to interact with the sensory space. Some of the items in Snoezelen rooms include black lights, bubble tubes, interactive panels, "soundbeans" designed for converting movements into sounds, projectors, vibration. The items are not cheap, but the rooms can be quite spectacular and wonderful!

A study by Novak *et al.* (2012) looked at outcomes associated with the introduction of a sensory room in an acute inpatient psychiatric unit. Both before and after each use of the room the researchers recorded self-reported levels of distress in users and disturbed behaviors reported by staff. In the room were various items, including weighted blankets. The study found that the sensory room was effective in reducing distress and disturbed behaviors and that weighted blankets seemed "particularly useful."

Helping patients getting weighted blankets covered by medical insurance

Some medical insurances in the U.S. will cover a weighted blanket.

For an insurance claim, patients will need a prescription from a doctor and a letter of medical necessity. The hospital OT can do a sensory evaluation for the letter of medical necessity. It should state that the blanket has helped them while in the hospital.

(See the medical insurance coverage section in Chapter 5 for more information.)

Chapter 5

Considerations/ Guidelines for Use

Can they create dependence?

No formal research has confirmed that users can become dependent on weighted blankets. However, people often find something that comforts them or causes them to feel more secure, and as a result they may prefer to use the item more often, like many children rely on a security blanket. For children there must be a treatment plan put in place by a trained therapist, and caregivers should be educated in their proper use and signs of distress.

Weighted blankets provide feelings of safety, calming, body regulation and grounding pressure to their users. They should *never* be used as a punishment or be forced on anyone. In fact, weighted blankets come with a responsibility; the caregiver or user should be instructed that the blankets are not for infant use nor should they be used by anyone who cannot remove them independently.

An additional concern is that studies designed to investigate the effectiveness of weighted vest use are being applied to the use of weighted blankets. Each is a different therapeutic tool and should be utilized accordingly.

So, what is the protocol for actual use? We will outline some of the most common strategies for weighted blanket use in this chapter.

How long to use the blanket?

In our study of OTs (Parker n.d.), we asked the question "How long do you advise keeping on the weighted blanket?" Many therapists reported that use depended on the individual child's response to the blanket. Answers ranged from ten minutes to up to one hour with removal of the blanket if it appeared uncomfortable in any way. Generally, therapists of older children recommended using the blanket according to the child's preferences. When using the blanket to decrease anxiety for medical procedures, therapists permitted use for the entire time of the procedure. Some reports state that the blanket's effect starts in three to five minutes, and some say it starts immediately. It has been reported that the blanket can reach the full effect in 15 to 20 minutes.

Temple Grandin (2006) writes in her book *Thinking in Pictures: My Life with Autism*: "Depending on the children's anxiety level, some will need access to deep pressure and swinging through the day, using it to calm themselves down when they become overstimulated."

A report by the Alberta College of Occupational Therapists Adhoc Task Force (2009) concludes that it "does not accept the OEQ's guideline of 20-minute maximum exposure. Both the tolerance of the child to the weighted blanket and the benefit of the weighted blanket must be considered when determining the length of time the weighted blanket should be applied. In the absence of evidence, the occupational therapist must ensure that the child is tolerating the weighted blanket well throughout his/her exposure to the weighted blanket." Occupational therapists must be integral members of the treatment team when weighted blankets are used as they can assist caregivers in determining the specific weight of a blanket on an individual basis.

Safety

Safety concerns are quite valid, since a boy and a baby have died using a weighted blanket.

In Québec, Canada, Gabriel was a nine-year-old with autism attending a school for disabled and special needs children. A teacher rolled him up in a 39-pound blanket with his face inside the blanket and left him there for up to 20 minutes.

A seven-month-old baby died in Webster Groves, Missouri. The baby was at a daycare where the blanket was placed on the lower half of his stomach, then the baby rolled over onto his stomach (Cambria 2014). The St. Louis medical examiner ruled the death as SIDS (sudden infant death syndrome). It isn't certain whether the weighted blanket was the cause of death. Regardless, a baby can't lift the blanket off himself or communicate that he has trouble breathing or finds the weight uncomfortable, painful, or upsetting.

The Ordre des ergothérapeutes du Québec released a purpose statement after the death of Gabriel to provide guidelines for safe use of weighted blankets by Occupational Therapists. This document can be viewed online, and provides detailed rules for how to ensure safe use of weighted blankets as a part of an occupational therapy plan. While we can't anticipate every instance that has a possibility of harm, here are guidelines for safety:

- Do not use the blanket on children under three years old because the filling inside can be a choking hazard.

- Do not ingest plastic beads. If swallowed, seek medical attention. They may cause gastrointestinal blockage.

- If the filling comes out of the blanket, clean it up immediately. Plastic pellets can be a slipping hazard, like walking on ball bearings.

- Do not put the blanket in the microwave since the filling is likely plastic. Instead, warm the blanket by putting it in the dryer for ten minutes.

- Do not roll up a person in a weighted blanket.

- Do not cover a person's head with a weighted blanket.

- Do not use it as a restraint. A person should be able to remove it by peeling it back much like one would with a comforter. I say "peel it back" because dead lifting the entire blanket from a prone position isn't practical.

- Do not use if there is a history of respiratory issues or a condition that may be compromised by putting weight on the body.

- Consult your doctor before use.

Drawbacks/concerns

Since weighted blankets are such a new concept, people may not necessarily understand how to handle them in everyday use, so they have concerns before and after they buy a weighted blanket.

The biggest concern is how to wash them. Once they know that they can be washed (assuming they have a washable filling), they ask how much stress it will be on their washer and dryer. I tell them that I wash my 34-pound queen-size in the washer then hang it to dry, and I have had no issues with the washer. But, I do have my husband take the wet blanket out of the washer for me because while wet, because it is too heavy for me.

Another option is to wash and dry it in a big washer and dryer at a laundromat. I have had a situation where a person with very sensitive allergies couldn't use that option because of the scented soaps and dryer sheets that others use, which would aggravate her allergies.

Some people do not like how hard it is to make the bed with such a heavy blanket to move around. I have had a couple of people exchange the blanket for a lighter weight for that reason.

Another concern is that the blanket will slide off the bed at night if a person turns over to their other side, which causes the blanket to shift. This has happened to me a couple of times, and it isn't fun putting a heavy blanket back on the bed while half asleep.

Some staff at hospitals and other institutions who use and launder the blankets heavily have found that the weight stresses the seams so that the blanket falls apart in part or entirely. This will vary by manufacturer.

Another concern is the cost of a weighted blanket. Cost can vary widely, but they are certainly not as cheap as a throw from Walmart. They cost a lot because they are very time-consuming to make since the most common method of making them is with individual pockets that get filled with weighting material and sewn one at a time. The cost will vary by manufacturer, depending on time spent and quality of materials and construction.

Medical insurance coverage

In the U.S, some medical plans will cover weighted blankets. However, some health insurance companies consider sensory integration therapy to be experimental and that the effectiveness of the therapy is unproven and therefore will not cover weighted blankets.

Since sensory processing disorder itself is not accepted as an official diagnosis in the *Diagnostic and Statistical Manual of Mental Disorders* (DSM-5), it's important to use terms which describe the dysfunctions that results from it. The therapist considers the functional impact of the SPD and identifies target goals and treatment areas. This information is shared with the treatment team, and the medical doctor or prescriber can create a prescription for a weighted blanket. Your OT may help to write a letter of medical necessity. Again, this letter must express that a weighted blanket has helped the patient while they are in the hospital.

Make sure the prescription doesn't state size, weight, or color since the weight that will work for you is likely different from what the doctor thinks, since doctors are not specialists on weighted blankets.

Weighted blanket companies do not process the claim since they are not licensed for that. You go through a durable medical equipment company (DME) to process the claim for you. You will have to hunt for one. They need to use the billing code, which is "E1399 Durable Medical Equipment, Miscellaneous." Once the claim is approved, the medical supply company contacts your chosen weighted blanket company to order the blanket.

It's not a fast process, but for some, they can get their blanket covered.

Your weighted blanket *may* be covered by medical insurance, but that does not mean it *will* be covered. Some plans are better at covering them, but even that is in constant flux, depending on changes to insurance and government legislation, and because insurance coverage differs by state.

For autism, for which a weighted blanket is standard medical equipment, over 30 states have mandated coverage for autism-related expenses. Does this mean weighted blankets must be covered? Is it recognized, according to the legislation, to be an autism treatment? To my knowledge, the coverage hasn't been tested yet. Also, the coverage is for *sensory integration disorder*, so technically, it isn't an autism expense. Yet, a sensory processing disorder is almost always present with autism. That fine wording can mean the difference between a "No" and a "Yes."

Sometimes, a state waiver or flex funds can also be used. A flexible spending account (FSA), maintained by your employer, lets you set aside pre-tax money for health-related expenses that your insurance may not cover, such as a weighted blanket.

As last I knew, TRICARE, the military's medical insurance, does not cover weighted blankets, even though they are such a help with PTSD.

Medicare does not cover them because coverage requires a separate billing code, which weighted blankets do not have yet. The Center for Medicare and Medicaid Services (2016) states on their website:

> Each year, in the United States, health care insurers process over 5 billion claims for payment. For Medicare and other health insurance programs to ensure that these claims are processed in an orderly and consistent manner, standardized coding systems are essential.

Note that Medicaid can be known by other names such as MassHealth in Massachusetts or Medical Assistance (M.A.) in Minnesota.

Their standard code system is the Healthcare Common Procedure Coding System (HCPCS, pronounced by its acronym as "hick picks"), which is a set of health care procedure codes based on the American Medical Association's Current Procedural Terminology (CPT). Weighted blankets do not yet have a HCPCS code, so when they are covered, it is with the code "E1399 Durable Medical Equipment, Miscellaneous." This code almost always requires pre-authorization from the insurer. If you have experience working with medical insurance, you could help others by applying for a new HCPCS code through the Centers for Medicare and Medicaid Services.

Place of residence can make a difference. National plans can be processed by any medical supply company in any state, regardless of where you live. Most states also have state-only plans, and if you have one of these plans, they will likely want the claim processed in your state, but that would vary among providers. With Medicaid, the claim has to be processed in your state.

There are a couple of deterrents to working with a DME. One, they usually have never heard of a weighted blanket. Two, the reimbursement amount from the insurer is sometimes less than the staff time to process the claim, so in essence, they may be spending more time on staff salary to process your claim than the actual dollar amount they would be earning. With persistence, though, some will process the claim for you.

For a medical claim, you will need supporting documentation that a weighted blanket will help, usually from a sensory profile done by an occupational therapist. Then, you will need a prescription from a doctor. Once the DME receives the documentation of medical necessity and the prescription, the insurance company will likely require prior authorization for the claim. Once the claim is approved, they order the blanket from a weighted blanket company.

You call a medical supply company, and they say, "Never heard of it. We don't carry those." Click. In my experience in getting weighted blankets covered, the responses can be courteous, rude, or curious. Persist. Tell each one that it is a medical equipment that is often covered, and they don't have to carry it in stock because it is ordered online. Do your homework, so you can tell them that you have a prescription and documentation. Tell them that it is covered under code E1399. Tell them that companies across the country have processed the claims successfully.

Even after a medical supply company says, "Yes," the rest of the staff may not know about it yet. Please do not get frustrated because it's a brand new thing for them. So, when you get to the initial person who said, "Yes," write down that person's name, so you can reference it later when you are working with the prior authorization folks.

Remember that you are not just the receiver of services, you are also the educator, so working as a team is important. You are on the leading edge, so the sell and the education are important.

Keep in mind that these companies usually pull from stock they have. But, since weighted blankets are typically custom-made then shipped directly to you, it will take a change in thinking for them. It's so easy; they could seem skeptical, but some are open to the idea.

This will take hours of your time and may take many months, but when you are looking at paying $100 or more outright, going the medical insurance route may be a good deal. Plenty of people have gotten them covered.

Out of curiosity, I called my medical insurance provider, and I learned how they want to see it covered (or not). The customer service representative said, "Say that again. What is it?" After he typed, he said, "Do you know the code for that?" He said it would require a manual review, meaning to send the prescription and documentation for them to review. He said to accompany it with a claim transmittal form found on my insurance website. He said to send copies instead of the originals. He reminded me that we have a health reimbursement account (HRA); I asked him in a couple of ways if I can use the HRA to pay for the weighted blanket if the claim gets denied.

As of this writing, a woman with the same insurance has gotten verbal approval for a weighted blanket for her son. The claim hasn't officially gone through the process with the medical supply company, so the jury is still out.

Which plan covers and which doesn't will change, so if your insurance doesn't cover it one year, they might the next or vice versa.

Chapter 6

Choosing or Making Your Own

Choosing a weighted blanket

For most people, a weighted blanket is a major purchase, so choosing the right one is important. There are many sizes, colors, patterns, fabric types, and weights to choose from. Some have removable weights, and some have an inner liner holding the weighting material, some have a covering on the blanket, and some have batting for warmth.

Almost all blankets are sold online and custom-made with your choice of fabric and weight. Finding the right one can be time-consuming, but worth the effort. Google doesn't always give every option on the first page, so it's worth doing a big of digging, and I'll tell you why.

Companies, including weighted blanket companies, spend a lot of time to get on the first page of a Google organic search ("organic" means actual search results that are not paid advertising). And rightfully so because while doing a search, most people don't explore beyond the first page. But, does that mean that the blanket and company you want is on the first page? Not necessarily. The weighted blanket maker on page two or page nine may be good at making weighted blankets, but not at getting on page one. They may not have the most stunning website, but wow, do they have great sewing machines! So, dig a little to learn about more options so you can land at the perfect weighted blanket for you.

Shopping for a weighted blanket is like choosing a car because there are so many variations in styles, colors, quality, and personal tastes.

The filling is an important consideration. Most weighted blankets are filled with a weighting material that consists of small pieces, then sewn into squares to distribute the weight evenly. Plastic pellets, also known as "poly pellets," are the most common way to add weight to the blanket. They also allow the finished blanket to be machine washed and dried.

Do not buy a weighted blanket weighted with organic materials such as popcorn, buckwheat hulls, dried beans, rice, or other organic materials. One liquid spill on the blanket makes the filling rot or sprout, and for the same reason, you cannot wash the blanket. Do not buy a blanket that contains lead shot because of the danger of lead poisoning.

> Lead poisoning occurs when lead builds up in the body, often over a period of months or years. Even small amounts of lead can cause serious health problems. Children under the age of 6 are especially vulnerable to lead poisoning, which can severely affect mental and physical development. At very high levels, lead poisoning can be fatal. (Mayo Clinic 2014)

There have been weighted blankets out there filled with lead shot even at a hospital, so make sure you know what the blanket is filled with before buying, including if you are buying it second hand. A hospital staffer I talked with was looking for another weighted blanket because they found out that their current blanket was filled with lead. They disposed of it immediately and did the "cleanup" needed when there was lead exposure.

Which fabric you use depends on your personal preference. Cotton or a polyester/cotton blend is the most common, and often the cheapest. People with autism will often have specific needs when it comes to fabric choice:

- plush like minky or fleece

- slippery like satin

- a grainy feeling like a cotton/polyester blend

- smooth like a high-count cotton sheet

- bumpy like ribbed or dotted chenille.

Color is another important choice. Color theory has been around for years, and there are no tried and true rules because personal preference plays a major role.

Keep in mind that autistic people typically experience visual stimuli to a higher degree than neurotypical people do. Choice of color intensity and hue can be important or, most often, necessary for them. High-contrasting colors can also be difficult, because it can make one or both of the colors seem to visually buzz, making the eyes feel painful. They may get a headache or feel upset so they want to get away from the contrasting colors *right now*.

Interior designer Denise Turner (2011) writes:

Researchers have found that autistic children's rods and cones (components of the eye) have changed due to chemical imbalances or neural deficiencies. Colors appear more vibrant to autistic children. Of the autistic children tested, 85% saw colors with greater intensity than non-autistic children. The color red for example, looks fluorescent and vibrates with intensity.

When it comes to choosing weighted blanket colors for the classroom, an interesting study found that red reduces a student's performance. Thalma Lobel's book *Sensation: The New Science of Physical Intelligence* (2014) tells of a team of American and German researchers headed by Andrew J. Elliot who set out to explore this connection between the color red and performance on achievement tests.

The student participants were given an anagram test. They were then divided into three groups, all with the same test, but the numbers at the top of the page were green, red, or black. The results were incredible—the subtle red text number had a dramatic effect. "Students who had a red number at the top of each page performed significantly worse... Similar studies had the same findings."

When choosing blanket colors for a child, I advise letting the child look on a weighted blanket maker's website to choose the colors he or she likes, so they can wrap themselves in colors that make them feel good. Children may have special color requests based on their interest, or they may just have a favorite color. As an example, a grandmother was buying a blanket for her grandson, and it had to be yellow and kelly green because he loved everything John Deere. When in doubt, ask the weighted blanket maker for samples, so your child can see the actual colors.

The choice of pattern is also worth noting for autistic people because they tend to spot patterns and can feel stressed when the pattern doesn't "match up." For example, a blanket pattern may not be perfectly aligned with the sewn squares or the fabric not cut exactly straight through a part of the pattern. The autistic person may be focusing on the incongruity over and over again, producing a stressed feeling. But, if the pattern is sewn perfectly, it may not be upsetting.

If you are buying a blanket as a gift for an autistic person, let them choose. If the person will not be choosing and you are in doubt about patterns, opt for solid colors.

Even when you have made the best choices for you, the blanket you receive may not be right for you. Weighted blanket makers strive to get the right blanket for you, but since a weighted blanket is a big investment, find out the company policies before you buy. Can you exchange the blanket for a different weight or size? Is there a restocking fee? Do you have to pay return shipping? Do you have to pay shipping to send out the second one? You can usually find out this information on their website; if not, send an email to find out their policies.

While there are weighted blankets available for shipping now, almost all weighted blankets are custom-made in your choice of fabric and weight. Since they are custom-made, keep production time in mind. Depending on how many orders the blanket maker has, it could take a week to three months to receive your blanket because usually they make orders in the order they receive them. Ask them where you are in the queue, so you have an estimate of how long it will take.

Predicting a specific day when the blanket will be ready is difficult because other factors come into play such as flu season or the seamstresses caring for children, parents, or grandchildren, or all of the above. Companies can sometimes be at the mercy of suppliers. For example, when I had my company, the longshoremen's union went on strike at the port of Los Angeles. This meant my suppliers couldn't get their product, so I ended up having to wait, and the customers had to wait.

Weighted blanket makers usually carry some stock fabrics, and when their supply gets low, they reorder as needed, but their supplier may not have what they need in stock at the time. Logic may dictate that they carry more fabric, but that could mean buying $1000 or more worth of fabric that just sits there. Even then, sometimes they will get an unanticipated run on a certain color or pattern, and they run out, even when they had extra in stock.

Blanket weight is an important choice, and there are no absolutes and no magic formulas to determine the weight. The guideline of 10 percent of body weight plus one pound has spread online. While the formula is not accurate for all people, it is a good starting point for children. For example, a seven-pound blanket for a sixty-pound child would be a good weight.

There are contradictions to the body weight rule. For example, Champagne *et al.* (2007) writes: "Body weight is generally not a factor influencing the amount of weight preferred." As an extreme example, a mother's 12-year-old, autistic son slept under his mattress, and she had to lie on the mattress so he could fall asleep. She bought a 40-pound queen-size blanket along with a 25-pound twin-size. She folded the queen in two and added the twin size. It worked for her son. Some people also need a super-heavy blanket, but for most, this weight would be unbearable.

Especially for adults, body weight isn't a reliable indicator of the person's desired weight on them. For example, I prefer a 34-pound queen on my bed, and I don't even weigh near 340 pounds. My weight has changed, yet the 34-pound queen still works for my sensory system. As another example, two women who are both 5'4" and weigh 140 pounds may like quite different weights.

In one case, a husband bought an 18-pound twin for his wife as a birthday present, which is in the normal range for most people. She found it way too heavy. She exchanged it for a ten-pound, which was perfect for her.

At hospitals, actually trying the weight on the patient and getting patient feedback on whether they want heavier or lighter is the best bet. It's much like pain—it's hard to objectively quantify.

In an interview, Dr. Anne Zachry, a pediatric occupational therapist, said:

> When it comes to using a weighted blanket with someone who has sensory processing issues, it is important to keep in mind that every individual's needs are unique. Research has not yet provided a set of guidelines, so it is necessary to make decisions related to the weight and size of the blanket on an individual basis.

When I had my weighted blanket business, Canadian organizations typically ordered lighter weights due to the child in Québec who had died at school from being rolled up in a weighted blanket, as mentioned in Chapter 5.

There is no way to be absolutely sure unless you try one. If you are considering buying one, make sure they have a return or exchange policy that honors returns and exchanges.

The blanket's size affects what weight you choose, and sometimes, blanket choice comes down to budget. For a child, the child size would make the most sense, but parents sometimes choose a twin instead, so as the child grows, it will still fit him. In the short term, the child size would be less expensive, but getting the twin will save money in the longer term—assuming that the child will not need a much heavier weight later.

When I had my weighted blanket company, I refined my weight chart based on what works for most people. Since I had a 100 percent exchange policy, I also knew what was too heavy or too light for people based on what people exchanged. For example, a 40-pound queen-size was exchanged for a lighter weight almost half the time.

I based our weight chart on what works for most people usually falling into the middle of a bell curve. Keep in mind that a ten-pound child-size will feel heavier than a ten-pound twin-size because in the twin, the filling is spread over a larger area. If you are unsure of what weight to order, err on the side of too light.

There are no standard sizes because each weighted blanket makers' sizes are different. However, there are some standard size ranges I read on blanket makers' sites in width and length:

- Child: 28"–34" wide by 50"–52" long

- Twin size: 39"–40" wide by 75"–76" long

- Double/Full: 54"–56" wide by 75"–82" long

- Queen: 60" wide by 82" long

Here is a weight chart of standard weights that I found work for most people.

	Child size	Twin	Double	Queen
Light	5 lb	10 lb	20 lb	22 lb
Most popular	7 lb	14 lb, 18 lb	27 lb, 32 lb	28 lb
Quite heavy	9 lb	22 lb, 25 lb	38 lb	34 lb, 40 lb

Weighted blanket makers strive to get an exact weight, but expect a small variation. Actual finished weight will vary based on who is filling the liner. Usually a pre-measured cup is used to fill the squares with the heavy filling. The weight of each cup can vary slightly according to who is filling the cup, but for a twin blanket, that person could be filling 190 squares, which could make the total weight vary by one to three pounds.

Fabric weight also varies. For example, cotton chenille weighs more than regular smooth cotton. It is difficult for a weighted blanket maker to take all fabric weights into consideration.

On a budget

Sometimes, a weighted blanket is financially out of reach, especially for families with an autistic child because their therapy expenses can be quite high.

One way to get a weighted blanket is to have family members get gift certificates toward all or a portion of the cost. Most weighted blanket makers offer a gift certificate option. Also, check online for coupons to use toward a blanket. Even if you don't see a coupon, contact the weighted blanket maker to ask for one and they will likely be able to help you.

People will sometimes contact a weighted blanket company to ask for a free weighted blanket. I have had people get angry with me for charging so much that people can't afford it. I have been blamed for taking advantage of special needs families by charging so much.

But, it costs money to make a weighted blanket: there is the cost of the materials and the biggest expense—paying people to make it. Also, if a weighted blanket maker doesn't make a profit, they can't pay the phone bill. Lastly, while most weighted blanket makers have a mission to help others with their blankets, almost all are in business to make a profit so they can support their own families. It's their job. I don't think any of them are millionaires yet, but I can guess that is not the aim of most.

Given all that, there are a couple of organizations where you can get a free weighted blanket, but you will have to wait a long time. Here are two organizations that make them free for children on the autism spectrum. Talk with the organizations to find out if your child is eligible.

The ISAAC Foundation makes and donates weighted blankets to children with autism in Washington. The child must reside in the ISAAC Foundation services area (Spokane, Stevens, Lincoln, Whitman and Kootenai Counties). Learn more at www.theisaacfoundation.org

Sharing the Weight, a non-profit in Iowa, donates weighted blankets. You can put yourself on their waiting list, which is quite long. You can also help. They need people in Ottumwa, Iowa area to sew these blankets and they need in-kind donations of fabric, thread, and plastic pellets. They also need money to ship the blankets. They need a lot of "boy" fabric since about five boy blankets are made to one girl blanket since boys are diagnosed with autism far more than girls. People outside of Iowa can help by making the "shells," which is sewing the blanket up to the point where it needs pellets. They also do something that sounds fun. They take their organization on the road. Bring a sewing machine to an Iowa event for a fun day of sewing with others like you, all to help children with autism. Learn more at www.sharingtheweight.org

Sewing your own weighted blanket

Another inexpensive option is to make your own. If you have a sewing machine, yet you are not a pro sewer, not to worry because it all involves sewing straight lines, and if they are not perfectly straight, it doesn't matter, though some people with autism may not like the irregular visual.

There are plenty of fabulous tutorials online, including on YouTube where you can see the actual construction taking place.

You will need:

- filling for the weight
- fabric (the width should be the width of the blanket required plus two seam allowances, and the length should be twice the length required plus four seams allowances)
- strong thread
- a scale
- a measuring cup or spoon.

Strong thread is important because the weight of the blanket will pull at the seams. If you are buying thread at a fabric store, choose thread that is described as "heavy" or "extra heavy" or made for denim or upholstery.

Blankets are usually made with square pockets to hold the beads, but who says you have to use straight lines? I think it would be fun to see weighted blankets with flowing, wavy lines instead of straight ones. Do be creative.

Basic instructions:

1. Cut two pieces of fabric to the size you want for the blanket, with a half-inch seam allowance.

2. Sew the two pieces of fabric together with the finished sides of the fabric facing each other.

3. Sew along three sides.

4. Turn the fabric inside out so the finished side of the fabric is facing out.

5. Sew channels along the length of the blanket leaving a half inch at the open end, which you will need to sew the blanket shut. The channels should be wide enough to pour in the filling, say four or five inches wide.

Next, calculate what weight you would like the blanket to be. Keep in mind that the weight will feel heavier or lighter depending on how much area the beads are spread out over.

1. Divide what you want the finished blanket to weigh by the number of squares you will be making. This is how much to pour in each measuring cup or spoon. However, the fabric weight should be considered for accuracy when measuring. For example, a textured fabric may be heavier than a cotton fabric. Different grades of fabric and even those with dyes versus natural colors can add weight. Subtle differences in the amount of fill in each pocket might add up when considering the total volume of the blanket. Remember to add the weight of the fabric to the total weight of your blanket.

2. When measuring on a scale, put the measuring cup on the scale and press "tare" or "zero."

3. Next, add the amount of plastic pellets to the measuring cup to get the weight you want.

4. Then pour the pellets into the channel so they fall to the bottom of the channel.

5. Do this for each channel.

6. Once you have pellets in all channels, sew across the blanket to seal the pellets in.

7. Repeat until all the squares are full.

8. When you have reached the end, sew the blanket shut by turning the seam allowance toward the inside of the blanket and sewing across.

While measuring the filling, be sure to make each measurement as accurate as possible. For example, if you are over by a half ounce in 50 squares, the blanket will be 25 ounces heavier.

A number of fillings can be used to provide the weight, such as plastic pellets, buckwheat hulls, BBs, popcorn kernels, rice, beans, glass beads, or pea gravel. Lead shot, while it has been used in the past, is absolutely *not* to be used. Lead is poisonous. It can cause severe developmental damage in children, and the poisoning is not quickly noticed because exposure can build up over time.

I don't recommend organic materials such as buckwheat hulls, popcorn, beans, or rice because with one liquid spill the blanket gets wet and the filling then can rot or sprout. If the blanket gets dirty, it can't be washed. As for BB pellets, they can also contain lead, but there are stainless steel ones coated with zinc or copper, with the copper currently being popular as an antimicrobial.

Glass pellets are an option. They are usually 1 mm or 2 mm wide, so they could possibly slip through the stitching if the stitching is not stitched closely. I recommend adding an outer covering so if beads do slip out, the outer covering will contain them. To find these, use the Google search term "glass pellets stuffing." They are called "stuffing" because they are commonly used for teddy bears and dolls, so the safety of these pellets is long known. The likelihood of them breaking into shards is minimal since they are so small. The benefit with these is that they provide extra pliability for the blanket, they are fairly quiet, and they make the blanket washable.

Pea gravel bears mentioning because it is so cheap to buy at any landscaping place. Pea gravel can have edges that could wear at the fabric. It could take a little longer to dry since it is somewhat porous.

River rock is smooth, so it may not wear as much on the fabric as pea gravel would. It will make the blanket somewhat lumpy, which some people may not like, but the multiple pressure points may feel good. It may ding up your dryer, so hang to dry.

Making the blanket with removable weights sounds like a good concept because the weights can be increased as a child grows and the shell of the blanket can be washed. If an adult will be using the blanket, interchangeable weights probably are not necessary.

Heavy chains can be a weighting material. The blanket can be sewn with long channels with a chain in each channel that is attached at each end. There is a weighted blanket company in Australia that uses this method.

The number one filling I recommend is plastic pellets. "Poly pellets" used to be the catchall name for plastic pellets, but Fairfield Processing has claimed the term "poly pellets" because they have been using it for so many years. Hence, the other poly pellet companies have had to change their websites and descriptions to something other than poly pellets, so "plastic pellets" is the new term for them. This is important for you because if you search with "poly pellets" you may not get all the companies you want to find in the search results.

You can find plastic pellets at Walmart, Michaels, Jo-Ann, and other places, often called "teddy bear stuffing." Keep in mind that the small one-pound or two-pound bags are more expensive than buying in bulk, but if you are making a lighter blanket for a child, this is a good option.

You can buy them in small quantities or in bulk on eBay or Etsy and from online companies that specialize in plastic pellets. Here are the top three:

- Craft Pellets (www.craftpellets.com)
- Fairfield Processing (www.fairfieldworld.com)

- Quality Plastic Pellets (www.qualityplasticpellets. com).

Plastic pellets can be made of different types of plastic. Two of the most common are high-density polyethylene (HDPE) and high-density polypropylene (HDPP). HDPE is typically white round pellets. HDPP is usually flatter and more see-through, though still tinged white.

In a weighted blanket or other craft project, keep in mind that the pellets will have some rustling noise. I had gotten a sample of low-density polyethylene (LDPE) because they are noticeably quieter, but they took up more room in the blanket squares, which made sewing difficult because of having to push even more of the pellets aside to sew the stitches to seal the square shut. In other words, more broken needles and more time spent.

Pellets can have variations in color, density, added chemicals, and more. Some are factory seconds and some are virgin plastic. While white or clear are the most common, they can come in many colors, and sometimes the colored ones are cheaper.

There are pellets that are extra heavy compared to the usual weight, yet are still a competitive price. You would be able to use fewer pellets to achieve the same weight.

Recycled pellets are sometimes an option, which can be cheaper. "Recycled" doesn't mean "dirty" because the plastic is melted at hundreds of degrees. There are also other types of plastic processing types available.

If you can find them, buy plastic pellets called "regrind." They are made into pellets from the leftovers from making plastic bags and other items, and since they are not using virgin plastic, they can be cheaper. Talk to your plastic pellet provider about what is best for your needs.

If you are buying large amounts, contact a pellet company: through them, you can buy a gaylord box, which is a huge box holding 1400 to 1600 pounds of pellets.

Postscript

Thank you for reading *The Weighted Blanket Guide*. Every effort has been made to provide up-to-date, unbiased, and accurate information. No information contained herein is a substitute for medical advice obtained by your physician.

If you have questions or suggestions or if you hear of new studies on weighted blankets, do let us know.

Connect with us

Eileen Parker
>   www.eileenparker.com
>   www.facebook.com/writereileen

Cara Koscinski, MOT, OTR/L, known as *The Pocket Occupational Therapist*
>   www.PocketOT.com
>   www.facebook.com/PocketOT

References

Alberta College of Occupational Therapy Adhoc Task Force (2009) *Commentary on l'Ordre des ergothérapeutes du Québec Position Statement on Use of Weighted Covers* [out of circulation].

American Psychiatric Association (2016) *Diagnostic and Statistical Manual of Mental Disorders (DSM)*. Available at www.psychiatry.org/psychiatrists/practice/dsm, accessed October 20, 2015.

Bundy, A.C., Shia, S., Qi, L., and Miller, L.J. (2007) "How does sensory processing dysfunction affect play?" *American Journal of Occupational Therapy 61*, 201–208.

Cambria, N. (2014) "Infant Death at Webster Groves Child Care Raises Concerns about Weighted Blankets." *St. Louis Post-Dispatch*, November 3, 2014. Available at stltoday.com/news/local/metro/infant-death-at-webster-groves-child-care-raises-concerns-about/article_922e0433-8931-5265-9d95-0aa1b5cd7faa.html?mobile_touch=true, accessed October 20, 2015.

Center for Medicare and Medicaid Services, The (2016) *HCPCS—General Information*. Available at www.cms.gov/medicare/coding/medhcpcsgeninfo/index.html, accessed on April 11, 2016.

Champagne, T., Mullen, B., and Dickson, D. (2007) *Exploring the Safety and Effectiveness of the Use of Weighted Blankets with Adult Populations*. Paper presented at the Annual Conference of the American Occupational Therapy Association. Available at http://sensorycalm.com.au/wp-content/uploads/2015/03/aota2007weighted_blanket_web_final_607.pdf, accessed October 20, 2015.

Champagne, T., Mullen, B., Dickson, D., and Krishnamurty, S. (2015) "Evaluating the safety and effectiveness of the weighted blanket with adults during an inpatient mental health hospitalization." *Occupational Therapy in Mental Health 31*, 211–233.

Cummings, K.S., Grandfield, S.A., and Coldwell, C.M. (2010) "Caring with comfort rooms: Reducing seclusion and restraint use in psychiatric facilities." *Journal of Psychosocial Nursing and Mental Health Services 48*(6), 26–30.

Edelson, S.M., Goldberg Edelson, M., Kerr, D.C.R, and Grandin, C. (1999) "Behavioral and Physiological Effects of Deep Pressure on Children With Autism: A Pilot Study Evaluating the Efficacy of Grandin's Hug Machine." *American Journal of Occupational Therapy* 53(2),145– 152. Available at https://newsinhealth.nih.gov/2007/february/docs/01features_01.htm, accessed February 29, 2016.

Grandin, T. (2006) *Thinking in Pictures: My Life with Autism.* New York, NY: Vintage Books.

Gringras, P., Green, D., Wright, B., Rush, C., *et al.* (2014) "Weighted blankets and sleep in autistic children: A randomized controlled trial." *Pediatrics* 134, 298–308. Available at http://pediatrics.aappublications.org/content/134/2/298, accessed October 20, 2015.

Hatch-Rasmussen, C. (n.d.) *Sensory Integration.* Available at www.autism.com/symptoms_sensory_overview, accessed October 20, 2015.

Lobel, T. (2014) *Sensation: The New Science of Physical Intelligence.* New York, NY: Atria Books.

Mayo Clinic (2014) *Lead Poisoning: Definition.* Available at www.mayoclinic.org/diseases-conditions/lead-poisoning/basics/definition/con-20035487, accessed October 20, 2015.

Mullen, B., Champagne, T., Krishnamurty, S., Dickson, D., and Gao, R.X. (2008) "Exploring the safety and therapeutic effects of deep pressure stimulation using a weighted blanket." *Occupational Therapy in Mental Health* 24, 65–89.

Najavitis, L. (2002) *Seeking Safety: A Treatment Manual for PTSD and Substance Abuse.* New York, NY: Guilford Press.

National Cancer Institute (2015) *Nerve Problems (Peripheral Neuropathy).* Available at www.cancer.gov/about-cancer/treatment/side-effects/nerve-problems, accessed April 4, 2016.

National Institutes of Health (NIH) (2007) *NIH News in Health,* February. Available at https://newsinhealth.nih.gov/2007/february/docs/01features_01.htm, accessed February 29, 2016.

Novak, T., Scanlan, J., McCaul, D, MacDonald, N., and Clarke, T. (2012) "Pilot study of a sensory room in an acute inpatient psychiatric unit." *Australasian Psychiatry 20,* 401–406.

Ordre des ergothérapeutes du Québec (2008) *OEQ Position Statement on the Use of Weighted Covers.* Available at http://cotbc.org/wp-content/uploads/OEQPositionStatement_WeightedCovers.pdf, accessed on April 7, 2016.

Parker, C. (n.d.) *OT Weighted Blanket Survey.* Available at www.eileenparker.com/ot-weighted-blanket-survey, accessed February 28, 2016.

Schaaf, R.C., Burke, J.P., Cohn, E., May-Benson, T.A., *et al.* (2014) "State of measurement in occupational therapy using sensory integration."*American Journal of Occupational Therapy 68*, e149–e153.

Sensory Processing Disorder Foundation (2016) *About SPD*. Available at www.spdfoundation.net, accessed April 4, 2016.

Sylvia, L.G., Shesler, L.W., Peckam, A.D., Grandin, T., and Kahn, D.A. (2014) "Adjunctive deep touch pressure for comorbid anxiety in bipolar disorder: Mediated by control of sensory input?" *Journal of Psychiatric Practice 20*, 71–77.

Teh, J.K.S., Cheok, A.D., Merritt, T., Peiris, R., *et al.* (n.d.) *Internet Pajama: A Mobile Hugging Communication System.* Available at http://citeseerx.ist.psu.edu/viewdoc/download?doi=10.1.1.83.98&rep=rep1&type=pdf, accessed October 20, 2015.

Turner, D. (2011) *Seeing Color Through Autistic Children's Eyes* [blog post]. Available at http://colorturners.blogspot.com/2011/03/color-autism.html, accessed October 20, 2015.

University of Miami School of Medicine Touch Research Institute (2013) "9 Incredible Reasons Why You Need to Give and Receive Hugs Everyday." *Collective Education.* Available at www.collective-education.com/tag/university-of-miami-school-medicine-touch-research-institute, accessed February 29, 2016.

U.S. Department of Health and Human Services (2006) *Federal Register Part 5: Rules and Regulations* 71(236), 71377–71427.

World Federation of Occupational Therapists (2011) *Statement on Occupational Therapy.* Available at www.wfot.org/Portals/0/PDF/STATEMENT%20ON%20OCCUPATIONAL%20THERAPY%20300811.pdf, accessed October 20, 2015.

Index

Page numbers in *italics* refer to tables.

actigraphy 17–18
Alberta College of Occupational
    Therapists Adhoc Task Force 78
Alzheimer's disease 24–25
American Academy of Pediatrics 17
American Medical Association 84
American Occupational Therapy
    Association 69
American Psychiatric Association 44, 82
antidepressants 52, 53–54
anxiety
    and autism 34–35
    in hospital settings 68, 69, 70, 72, 73
    use of weighted blankets to reduce
        16, 23, 67, 69, 70, 72, 73, 78
associations, positive and negative 40, 42
autism
    anxiety and 34–35
    male/female prevalence 96
    use of massage 50
    use of weighted blankets 16, 18,
        23–24, 55–56, 83, 89, 90–91,
        92, 96
Autism Research Institute 39
Ayres, Anna Jean 38–39, 44

behavioral therapy 65, 67
billing codes 82, 83, 84, 85, 86
bipolar disorder 25–26
borderline personality disorder (BPD)
    27, 67
Brain Research Institute, UCLA 39
brain, the 20–21, 23–24, 39, 48, 52–57, 64
breathing, deep 60, 62
Bundy, A.C. 45
Bush, President George W. 66

calming techniques 60, 62, 71, 73, 74, 78
Cambria, N. 79
Center for Medicare and Medicaid
    Services, The 83, 84
central nervous system (CNS) 20–21,
    27, 53, 56
Champagne, T. 61, 69, 70, 92
chemical dependency 27, 67, 68
chronic pain 16, 20–22, 55
cloves, use of 38
cognitive therapy 65
Cokato Charitable Trust 24
Coldwell, C.M. 73
color issues 73, 74, 89–90, 91
comfort/multisensory rooms 73–75
cortisol 50
Craft Pellets 100
Cummings, K.S. 73

deep breathing 60, 62
deep pressure 16, 25–26, 27, 35, 41,
    48–49, 61
    see also massage
dementia 24–25, 52
dependence issues 77–78
depression 51
    antidepressants 52, 53–54
*Diagnostic and Statistical Manual of
    Mental Disorders*, DSM-5 44, 82
Dickson, D. 69, 92
dopamine 48, 56
durable medical equipment companies
    (DMEs) 82, 84, 85
dyspraxia 45–46

Edelson, S.M. 49
Elliot, Andrew J. 90
employment issues 42, 46–47, 64
endorphins 51
exercise 51, 59, 63

Fairfield Processing 100
fibromyalgia 16, 20–22, 50
Field, Tiffany 49
fight-or-flight response 23, 46, 50
flexible spending accounts (FSAs) 83
folk medicine 37–38
Food and Drug Administration (FDA)
    52, 56

ginger, use of 37–38
Google 87–88, 99
Grandfield, S.A. 73
Grandin, Temple 5, 34–35, 78
Gringras, P. 17
grounding 62, 67

Hatch-Rasmussen, C. 39
health reimbursement accounts (HRAs)
    86
Healthcare Common Procedure Coding
    System (HCPCS) 84
hearing, sense of 40
hospitals 65–73
    restraint reduction 66–71
    use of weighted blankets 16, 26,
        27–28, 32, 71–73, 73–75, 81
hugs 29, 48–49, 61
hyper-responsivity 26, 65
hypo-responsivity 65

infants 77, 79, 80
infection control 71–72
insomnia 16, 19
insula (insular cortex) 20–21, 54–55, 57
insurance see medical insurance
internet pajamas 49
ISAAC Foundation 96

Kalla Lily Salon and Spa 50

lead poisoning 88, 99
Leonhart, Angie Balzarini 27–28
limbic system 48
Lobel, Thalma 90
Lycra 61

McKean, Tom 35
magnetic resonance imaging (MRI) 48,
    52, 55
massage 16, 21, 49–51, 63
Mayo Clinic 88

Medicaid 83–84
medical insurance 14, 68, 75, 82–86
Medicare 83–84
meltdowns 24, 43, 47, 60
mental illnesses, use of weighted
    blankets for 25–28, 65–71
menthol 56
mind–body connection 51, 52
mindfulness 51
Mireau, Clarissa 67–68
morphine 51
mosquitos 52–53
MRI see magnetic resonance imaging
Mullen, B. 14, 69, 92
multiple sclerosis 50
multisensory rooms 73–75
Mystery of Pain, The (Nelson) 20, 21

Najavitis, Lisa 62
National Cancer Institute 21
National Institutes of Health (NIH) 48
Nelson, Doug 20, 21
neuroscience 52–57
New Freedom Commission on Mental
    Health 66
New Science of Physical Intelligence, The
    (Lobel) 90
Novak, T. 75

occupational therapists/therapy (OT)
    16, 27–28, 59–65, 67, 84
    definition 59–61
    how weighted blankets are used 23,
        61–62, 78–79, 79–80
    and sensory integration therapy 15,
        38–39, 44, 62–63, 82
    and SPD 39, 44, 45, 62–65, 74
    use of massage 51
Ohio State University 52
Ordre des ergothérapeutes du Québec
    (OEQ) 78, 79–80
organic materials 88, 99
OT see occupational therapists/therapy
oxytocin 48, 61

Parker, C. 14, 18, 78
patterns, matching 18, 90
pellets
    glass 99
    plastic 73, 80, 88, 99, 100–102
physical therapists/therapy 16, 51

Piehowski, Stacie 50
post-traumatic stress disorder (PTSD)
    16, 23, 65, 83
pressure suits 35
professional settings 59–75
    comfort/multisensory rooms 73–75
    hospitals *see* hospitals
    medical insurance *see* medical
        insurance
    occupational therapy *see* occupational
        therapists/therapy
Prohofsky, Gretchen 26, 68–69
proprioceptive system 28, 34, 40, 55, 64
psychotherapy 73
PTSD *see* post-traumatic stress disorder

Quality Plastic Pellets 101
quiet rooms 28
quilts 31–34

Regions Hospital 26, 27–28, 68–69
regulation, of the body 20, 24, 45, 46,
    48, 49–50, 70, 77
    self-regulation skills 26–27, 28, 61
relaxation techniques 27, 28, 49, 50, 60,
    62, 73–75
restless legs syndrome (RLS) 21, 22
restraints 17, 25, 26, 66–71, 80

safety concerns 5, 72–73, 79–80
safety sitters 26, 68
St. Joseph's Hospital 67–68
Schaaf, R.C. 47
selective serotonin reuptake inhibitors
    (SSRIs) 53–54
self-injury 27, 67, 71, 73
self-regulation skills 26–27, 28, 61
seniors 24–25
sensory integration therapy (SI) 15,
    38–39, 44, 62–63, 82
sensory integrative dysfunction *see*
    sensory processing disorder
sensory over-responsivity (SOR) 26, 65
Sensory Processing Disorder
    Foundation 24, 44
sensory processing disorder (SPD)
    23–24, 26, 42–45, 67, 68, 68–69, 83
    comorbidity 43, 46
    occupational therapy and 39, 44, 45,
        62–65, 74, 82

problems resulting from 45–48
    research 43–44
    sensory integration therapy and 15,
        38–39, 44, 62–63
sensory profiles 84
sensory rooms 73–75
sensory system 38–45, 52–57, 64
serotonin 53, 56
Sharing the Weight 96
sleep issues 16, 17–20, 19–20, 25
smell, sense of 65
Snoezelen rooms 74–75
SPD *see* sensory processing disorder
special education/needs 28–30, 47,
    74, 95
spirituality 67
squeeze machines 5, 34–35
Stanford University 55
State Trait Anxiety Index (STAI-10)
    69, 70
stress hormones 46, 49, 50
substance misuse 27, 67, 68
sudden infant death syndrome (SIDS) 79
survival instinct 23, 42, 46, 50, 64
Sylvia, L.G. 25–26

tactile system 23, 28, 34, 35, 41, 45, 48,
    61, 63
taste, sense of 55, 65
Teh, J.K.S. 49
Therafin Corporation 35
Thinking in Pictures: My Life with Autism
    (Grandin) 78
touch, problems with 29, 48, 54
Tracy, Susan E. 59
trauma 27, 67, 73
TRICARE 83
Turner, Denise 89

UCLA Brain Research Institute 39
University of Miami School of Medicine
    Touch Research Institute 48–49, 49
U.S. Department of Health and Human
    Services 66

vestibular system 40–41, 64
visual system 40, 89

warmth 13, 87

weighted blankets
  choosing or making your own 87–102
    on a budget 95–96
    choosing 87–95
    sewing your own 96–102
  cleaning 71–72, 80–81
  color 89–90, 91
  concept 31–35
    old meeting the new 31–32
    origins 34–35
    others' stories 32–34
  considerations and guidelines for use
      77–86
    dependence 77–78
    drawbacks and concerns 80–81
    length of time to use 78–79
    medical insurance 82–86
    safety 5, 72–73, 79–80
  cost 81, 85, 95–96
  deaths when using 79
  definition 13–14
  free 95–96
  freezing 73
  how they work 37–57
    deep pressure 48–49
    massage 49–51
    neuroscience 52–57
    problems resulting from SPD
        45–48
    sensory system 38–45
  materials used 15, 70, 71–72, 73, 80,
      88–89, 95, 98–102
  patterns 90
  professional settings 59–75
    comfort/multisensory rooms
        73–75
    hospitals see under hospitals
    medical insurance see medical
        insurance
    occupational therapy see
        occupational therapists/
        therapy
  size 92, 93–94, 94
  use 14–30
    Alzheimer's/dementia/seniors
        24–25
    anxiety see under anxiety
    autism see under autism
    chronic pain and fibromyalgia
        20–22
    mental illnesses 25–28

sleep 17–20
  special education 28–30
  warmth 13, 87
  weight issues 5, 15, 18, 69, 70, 79, 81,
      82, 92–95, 94, 100
weighted vests 29, 70, 77
Wenk, Gary 52–57
World Federation of Occupational
    Therapists 59–60

Lightning Source UK Ltd.
Milton Keynes UK
UKOW06f0209040616

275581UK00001B/69/P